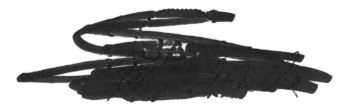

CLAWHAMMER

CLAWHAMMER

Sam
Llewellyn

POCKET BOOKS

New York   London   Toronto   Sydney   Tokyo   Singapore

This book is a work of fiction. Names, characters, places, and incidents are either products of the author's imagination or are used fictitiously. Any resemblance to actual events or locales or persons, living or dead, is entirely coincidental.

 POCKET BOOKS, a division of Simon & Schuster Inc.
1230 Avenue of the Americas, New York, NY 10020

Originally published in Great Britain in 1993 by Michael Joseph Ltd.

Library of Congress Cataloging-in-Publication Data

Llewellyn, Sam, 1948–
    Clawhammer / by Sam Llewellyn.
      p.   cm.
    ISBN 0-671-78989-9
    1. Political crimes and offenses—Fiction. 2. Poets—Fiction.
I. Title.
PR6062.L39C57   1994
823'.914—dc20   93-8241
                                                                CIP

First Pocket Books hardcover printing January 1994

10   9   8   7   6   5   4   3   2   1

POCKET and colophon are registered trademarks of
Simon & Schuster Inc.

Interior design by Allen Rosenblatt

Printed in the U.S.A.

To D. X. Shnaider

CLAWHAMMER

1

*I*T WAS HOT ON THE VERANDA, THAT LAST NIGHT. IT WAS ALWAYS hot. Africa stretched away, baked dry, a thousand miles in all directions. Rhydian Walters, my sister's husband, had his famous guitar on his famous knee. Camilla, my sister, was sitting in a rocking chair under a kerosene lantern spinning with moths, sewing nametapes on to the gray flannel shirts of her sons.

And of course we had been talking about the sea.

Rhydian always talked about the sea when departures were imminent. Tonight I was getting ready to take his sons, my nephews, back to school in England. He had talked his way from Boston north and east to Penobscot Bay, Maine, his home. "Make your mouth water," he was saying. "All that snow, rain. Precipitation City."

"You hated the rain," said Camilla, without looking up. Rhydian was a poet, if you can call semiretired country and western heroes poets, as well as being violently practical. Camilla was just violently practical.

Rhydian grinned at her, the grin that had propelled him to

number one in the country chart with "The Alleluia Tree," one of the last records he had made before he had joined the educational charity PloughShare and come gardening in Ethiopia. He hit a chord on his guitar, pulled a lick out of the top three strings, and sang:

> You're so down to earth
> (I hate ter
> Say this, babe)
> You make a crater . . .

Camilla threw a gray shirt at him. He hit another chord. The guitar neck broke with a sound like a brick thrown into a piano.

Rhyd picked up the neck of the guitar and examined the break. He said, "Ants." He began to laugh.

I looked at Camilla. Her blue eyes were shadowed by her strong bones. Her hair was bound back in a yellow ponytail. Her face was solemn. It was solemn because Rhyd was a guitar addict, and guitars are hard to find in the Ethiopian semi-desert. That must have been the reason. Camilla did not believe in omens.

Rhyd said, "Studio time." He got up. "You two want to come down?"

"Sure," I said.

Camilla held up a shirt, and shook her head. We walked into the house to the earth-floored mud-walled back room where Rhyd kept his Teac portastudio.

He shoved a white felt Stetson on his head and sat down behind the synthesizer. The room filled with the heavy, lurching stomp of a bass. He laid a synthesizer track over the bass, then reached for the curly horned Gibson mandolin hanging on the wall. I sat and listened, sweating gently in the heat.

In the U.S.A., Rhyd had been a large scale country and western hero. He still wrote a lot of songs, and he sent the demos home to his publishers and manager and friends and relations the way other people wrote letters. He played the mandolin track, cross-picking, one take only, solid and precise, the way he did everything. He said, "Vocals next. Let's have a beer."

I went to the solar-powered fridge he had manufactured from the bowels of an ex-military freezer and took two beers from beside the remains of a Christmas pudding. Christmas had been a week ago. It was too hot in the studio. I said, "Coming out?"

He said, "I have to finish this tonight. I want to get some tapes ready for you to mail."

I went back out to the veranda and talked to Camilla. For the sake of coolness we talked about England; the cottage behind Pulteney in Devon where we had once lived together and I lived still. At two in the morning, I went to bed. All night as I thrashed under the mosquito net I could half hear the electric pulse of the bass thumping faintly in the walls.

Eventually I fell into a sweaty sleep. In the morning, the light crept through the curtains and lay on the beaten-earth floor like puddles of white-hot iron.

And the last day began.

The village lay in a bowl of brown hills. High on the slopes, sheets of naked rock caught the heavy glare of the sun and shone like plates of metal, hurting the eye.

Lower down the slopes, stone walls wandered across bluffs and into dry valleys. They went for miles, those walls. Unless you already knew, it was hard to work out their purpose. Once, the people of the village said, there had been cattle up there, flocks of sheep and wheeling hawks. That was before the people of the village had cut the trees for firewood, and the cattle had torn the last of the vegetation from the ground, so there was nothing to hold the soil. Then the rains had washed the soil into the river that in times of flood ran down the boulder-strewn wadi in the center of the village. When the soil had gone, the cattle had died. Nowadays, up above the walls on the mountainside, you could find their bones, and a lot of lizards. In the bad times there had been few lizards, because most of them had been eaten.

It was Rhyd who had suggested the building of the walls. The people of the village had nodded politely and done nothing, partly because they knew that all white men were mad, and partly because they were too hot and too little nourished to do anything requiring more effort than nodding politely.

So Rhyd had gone up there himself, and Camilla with him. And with the sun bouncing off their fair Anglo-American heads, they had started to build.

I climbed out of bed, padded across the beaten-earth floor to the kitchen. Joe and Harry were there at the table, eating millet porridge. Joe was thirteen, long faced like his father, beginning to be bleary eyed. "Morning, jailer," he said.

His brother Harry was eleven, and therefore still of an age to be bright in the mornings. He looked like a blondish cherub planning mayhem. "When are we off?" he said.

"Lunchtime. Can't you wait?"

"It's the lizards," he said. "Got to release the specimens."

Harry's private life was conducted in a sea of lizards, inside and outside a collection of tin-can vivaria. There were plenty of lizards around nowadays. Since Rhyd and Camilla's arrival, they had gone out of fashion as a food item.

I took a cup of coffee to the veranda, sat down on a bamboo chair in the shade of the morning glories growing up the posts that supported the roof, and watched the swallows hawking for insects over the Alleluia Tree.

The second day of Rhyd and Camilla's wall building, a couple of men had arrived; stick-thin men with big cloaks the color of unbleached flour. They had laughed a lot, pointed, and gone home to the village of clay houses in the dust caldron of the valley.

The wall building went on for five months. Camilla spent ten days in bed with sunstroke. Rhyd lost twenty pounds.

At the beginning of the sixth month, it rained.

Normally, the water came straight down the valleysides in a sheet, a gray-brown torrent that filed away topsoil, poured into the dry wadi, and hurled itself in a welter of scum toward the Blue Nile.

This time, something new had happened.

When the sheet of water hit the base of the wall, it began to flow sideways, following the line of stones. At the wall's lowest point, Rhyd had gouged a dewpond from the hillside. The dewpond filled with water. The overflow followed the base of another wall into another channel. The channels zigzagged down the hill like the tracks of a cautious skier. The whole side of the valley was embroidered with silver threads of water.

In shallow pools and on the downhill side of the dewponds, where the soil was damp with seepage, Camilla planted little green seedlings that she had grown in the shady place behind their hut. Then Rhyd went to the old men in the village, and engaged in long, elliptical conversations.

I finished the coffee and looked at the topmost wall. Above it the mountain was yellow and brown, glinting with boiler-plates of rock. Below the wall, it was green. Trees grow fast in big heat if there is water around their roots. And fruit bushes grow in the shade of trees, and yams and other tubers under the fruit bushes. People in the village had become unused to the idea of hunger.

Up on the ridge, where what passed for the road crossed the lip of the valley, a thread of smoke cut the clear blue sky and a windscreen flashed in the sun. To navigate the ruts and boulders on the roads, you needed four-wheel-drive vehicles. The only people who had four-wheel-drive vehicles were soldiers. Ethiopia was full of soldiers nowadays: gangs of farmboys with Kalashnikovs, jockeying for position in what overwrought Western journalists were calling an emerging African democracy.

Rhyd arrived with a cup of coffee. He sat down. He said, "Are you coming down to the workshop?"

I said, "We've finished the pump. I should pack."

He said, "That was a big help." His eyes said: Hang around, don't go, help with the work. But Rhyd knew by now that I was not a stayer.

I said, faintly awkward, "I should get back to it."

He nodded. He had a face like an outcrop of rock, a butte of a jaw, a crag of a nose; sandstone-red sunburn with sleepless black circles under his eyes. There was something gaunt and fleshless about his face that morning, as if he had taken a look at the future and knew what had to happen.

Or perhaps it was just that he was missing his guitar, and thinking about missing his sons.

I said, "I'll send you another guitar."

"Oh." He grinned the famous grin, as if he had just woken up. "Guitar, yeah." He paused. Then he said, "I'm glad you're getting the kids out of here."

I said, "What do you mean?"

He waved at the brown hills. "Too many guns," he said. He handed me a brown paper package. "Tapes," he said. "Don't forget to post them."

He tipped the dregs of his coffee into the soil of a tin can in which a gourd was growing. "Back to the coalface." He walked down the veranda steps, across the beaten earth to the workshop.

The workshop was where he ran a blacksmithing and metalwork service, converting military debris into farm machinery. We had been making a pump from a wrecked fire engine. There was a need for pumps since the building of the walls, because the water table had risen to the point where the wells were functioning again.

In the sun, the ground was the bright dun of a lion's flank. Under the Alleluia Tree, it was ink-black with shadow.

The Alleluia Tree was a giant, flat-topped acacia. When Rhyd had arrived, its shadow had been the only patch of shade in the whole hot landscape. It was the center of the village, a meeting place and resthouse for people and animals. The village's important houses looked out onto its gnarled trunk. Rhyd had been allocated a site there in his third year in the village. And it was there that he had sited the workshop, because it was there that the workshop's customers met.

When Rhyd passed into the workshop compound, twenty voices rose in greeting.

The thing you noticed about Rhyd and Camilla was that you hardly noticed them at all. Nowadays, Rhyd was the village blacksmith and Camilla was the district nurse and horticultural adviser. They had other connections, about which they did not talk much. Nobody survived long in the intricate clan systems of the mountains unless they understood the politics. I could have asked them, if I had been interested. But I studied poetry instead of politics, and birds instead of agriculture.

This time, I had been making watercolor paintings of bustards down in the riverbed. The bustards were another thing that had come back since Rhyd and Camilla. The paintings were dry. I went to my room and packed them up sandwiched between boards. I walked down into the village. The sun was high, the houses still. A child watched from a doorway. I went into the house of Esias the silversmith.

The house smelled of cumin and hot metal. Esias squatted in the corner, tapping with a hammer at a sheet of raw silver on a tiny anvil. I watched as the sheet became a curve, the curve a bowl. When Esias was ready, he looked up. "You go," he said. He reached for the spidery coffeepot standing by the little furnace.

Over my visits to the village Esias had become a friend. We barely spoke each other's languages, but he seemed appreciative of my paintings, and I admired his skill with his hammer and his little anvil, his sheets of silver and his semiprecious stones.

Esias said, "It is a good time to go." His face was grim, his eyes heavy on either side of the thin-bridged nose. "There is fire in the hills."

"Fire?"

"All will be melted," he said. His eyes shifted away from mine. He drained his coffee and clasped my hand.

I said, "What do you mean?"

He shook his head. He still would not look at me. "You must go," he said, and towed me to the door.

I walked up to the house, out of the sun and into the black shade of the Alleluia Tree. I did not understand, but in the village I was used to not understanding. I climbed the veranda steps, went to my room, sat down in the canvas chair. The bead curtain on the door rattled. Camilla was there.

She was my oldest and dearest friend. My mouth was suddenly dry with nerves. I could feel thousands of miles of hostile emptiness pressing in. I said, "Esias is worried."

She smiled, the electric smile. Her face was thinner than formerly, the brown skin stretched tight over the high cheekbones. "Old Esias," she said. "What does he know?"

"He is talking about fire in the hills," I said.

The smile went. "There has been a civil war," she said. "It's not surprising that people talk like that."

I nodded. She was only five years older than me, but she had more or less brought me up. Even now, if she told me something was all right, I believed her.

"So you get out of civil war, and into . . . other things," she said.

"What do you mean?"

Her smile had a wry twist. "Freedom," she said. "Democracy. Everyone cheers. But you get surprise gifts in the packet."

"What are you talking about?" Camilla and Rhyd's central idea had always been that practical assistance was more important than politics.

"There comes a time when you can't not get involved."

I said, "So you're involved."

She smiled, brightly. "We're all involved."

"In what?"

She said, "You're going back to England. Tell people what you've seen." She looked at her watch. "Come on."

She hugged me. I hugged her back. I knew of old that if Camilla wanted to protect you from something, you stayed protected.

She said, "Bring the boys back?"

"Next holidays."

We smiled at each other. Against her brown skin her eyes were the genuine periwinkle blue. We both knew, in the way that people who have lived together for the first twenty years of their lives know, that under the smiles we were worried.

Except that she knew what we were worried about. And I had no idea.

2

WHEN WE TOOK THE BAGS ONTO THE VERANDA, THE PLUME OF smoke was no longer rising from the pass. But high up, where the boulder-strewn track began its long hairpins, another windscreen flashed in the sun.

"Boys," I called, "you ready?"

Harry appeared from his room, hands in the pockets of his khaki shorts, looking cool so as not to look sad. Joe came out of one of the narrow streets of brown houses, carrying a spear, trailing a bunch of black children. They were talking. Joe was a linguist, like his father. He salaamed. They salaamed back. He brought the spear on to the veranda. As he mounted the steps, the young warrior's dignity left him. He became a gawky schoolboy holding an African curio.

"Here comes Derek," said Harry.

High in the east, a silver mote hung in the blue. The buzz of an engine tore the vast silence. Rhyd came out of the workshop and strode across the beaten earth under the Alleluia Tree. Behind him, inside the compound gate, African faces were limned with the blue glow of a welding torch. He hugged the boys. "Take it easy," he said. "Give our love to Blighty."

"It's a long way to Tipperary," said Harry. Joe grinned. England was the war zone, as far as the boys were concerned. "Out of Eden and back to the trenches."

It was a time-honored formula that took the place of the unsayable things they all wanted to say. I looked away. I was outside the circle: the uncle, the jailer. I watched the silver dot become a cross, then a high-wing Cessna airplane. We walked to the strip beside the riverbed. The plane skimmed in, blew gritty dust over us, taxied back. I kissed Camilla's lean brown cheek.

She said, "Come back soon," and drilled me with the eyes. I grinned to hide a wave of depression, caused partly by leaving her and partly by the prospect of flying. Then I shook a lot of hands, climbed into the plane and checked the boys' straps.

Derek was the pilot. He was a Kikuyu from Kenya, and he knew the boys well. Everyone said, "Jambo," with great fluency, and a choke in the voice. The inside of the plane smelled of petrol and hot plastic. The engine howled. Dust billowed from under the wings as we tore down the baked-earth runway. The land dropped away, taking my stomach with it. I shut my eyes surreptitiously.

Derek said, "We got plenty fuel. We take a look around, okay?"

"Fine," said Joe. Joe would rather fly around in airplanes than eat.

"So up we go," said Derek. "You ever seen it from high up? Like a green emerald in a golfing bunker, I promise you."

He took us up in a big, lazy spiral that brought my heart to my mouth and cold sweat to my palms. A couple of olive-drab trucks were trailing dust into the village from the direction of the pass. They would be the ones whose windscreens had flashed earlier. The valley became a brown bowl. Sharply outlined by the serpentine wriggle of stone walls across hillsides was the Zulu shield of green Rhyd and Camilla had brought into being. In the center of the shield was the clay maze of the village with the dusty ribbon of the landing strip. "So that what your mam and dad done," said Derek.

I looked down into the green jewel.

In the middle of the maze, next to the dark green of the Alleluia Tree, a chip of ruby glowed. I frowned. There should be no ruby.

The chip flared, became orange. The orange was edged with black smoke.

"Down," I said. It came out as a croak.

Derek looked at me, eyes wide and white in his glossy black face. Then he shoved his stick forward, and Harry was screaming a fairground scream in the back seat as we became weightless in the dive.

The Cessna plummeted out of the sky like a stooping hawk. I shut my eyes. The cabin filled with the howl of wind. I leaned over to Derek. I opened my eyes and yelled in his ear, "Bank left at the bottom!"

He nodded. His teeth were bared. Muscles were working at the corners of his jaw. When you spend time in the poorest countries in Africa, you learn that sudden gouts of flame seldom mean good news for anybody.

The jewel grew. It became a toy bungalow, with flames streaming from the thatch. Two toy lorries were parked in the tennis-racket–shaped shade of the Alleluia Tree. Toy soldiers were milling around, growing as the Cessna dropped, forming a horseshoe. My mouth was dry with fear, and not only of airplanes.

Two figures came out of the front of the bungalow, fast, stumbling. When they looked up at the noise of the plane their faces were white. They were wearing the clothes Rhyd and Camilla had been wearing. They raised their arms in the air and faced the horseshoe of soldiers. Then something happened to them, and they fell down on the beaten earth between the bungalow and the Alleluia Tree.

The sweat on my body turned to ice.

Joe said, "I can't see."

Harry said, "Nor can I."

Derek said something that sounded like spitting. I heard his foot stamp on the rudder pedal, the groan of the airframe as he banked left, pulling away from what was happening down there, hiding it from the boys. The Alleluia Tree's canopy whisked under the wing.

Something hit the airplane with a crash. Suddenly there was a round hole in the windscreen, starred at its edges. Derek turned his plane's tail to the bungalow and flew away.

"Back," I said. My vision was blurred. I could not believe what I had just seen.

Derek said, "We got the kids. We go back, we all get it."

Joe said, "What's happening?"

Harry said, "It's not fair. I couldn't see."

I said, "There's nothing to see. Off we go, my dears."

Then I put my face in my hands.

We landed at a mission a hundred miles to the northeast. Joe said, "What's going on?"

I tried to smile reassuringly. But the muscles of my face were numb, and I could only say, "I don't know," with a mouth that did not seem able to pronounce the words.

"Some balls-up," said Harry. He looked anxious, too. He was trying to make it all right with something like a joke.

I said, "I've got to go and have a look at something. You'd better wait here."

Normally, they would have objected. They had seen nothing. But they knew things were not normal.

A couple of nuns were walking toward us, gray and black, like hooded crows. I had met them before: Sister Angela and Sister Dervla. I went to meet them. I told them what had happened. Their wrinkled brown faces turned gray, and they closed their eyes.

The reek of avgas was sharp as we refueled the Cessna. Then we took off into a sky now heat hazed with noon, wheeled over the T-shirted boys and their gray and black escort, and bumped back to the village.

Derek aimed the Cessna at a high, hot ledge. Rocks flashed in front of my face. When the plane was still and the dust had drifted away, I slipped a portable two-way radio into my pocket and jumped onto the ground. Sweat ran stickily off me as I clambered up to the ridge. It occurred to me vaguely that the people in the trucks might still be in the village. The thought seemed separate from its consequences. I went on.

I slithered down the bare upper slopes in a cloud of dust. Below the walls, the green ground gave off a loud whirr of insects. There did not seem to be any trucks any more. There was only a black wisp of smoke rising into the still air, and the baa of a rangy sheep from the paddocks on the edge of the village. And from the narrow brown streets, another sound, high and shrill, rising and falling like a siren.

I came through the widest street of the village and into the patch of beaten earth at the center. Grim-faced children watched big eyed from the safety of dark doorways. My knees were jellied with fear.

The Alleluia Tree still stood, but its leaves were gone. It was black and gaunt, raising naked arms at the hot blue sky. Its shade was thin and lacy, a network of spidery black lines on the yellow ground.

The women were in what remained of its shade, looking at what remained of the bungalow. They were squatting on the ground with their flour-colored cloaks piled on their heads, keening the dead. The men were standing in front of them, watching the ashes as if they expected something to happen.

Nothing was going to happen.

Straw and timber burn quickly when you fire an RPG into the middle of them. Clay will crumble. There was a single charred pole standing like a grave marker in the middle of a square of soft ash. There was a harsh and bitter smell of burning.

The crowd parted in front of me. I walked across the beaten earth to what had been the veranda. I was holding my breath. There was no reason. There was nothing to see.

One of the men in the crowd came forward. He was old, maybe forty-five, with a white beard and a high forehead and a long, narrow-bridged nose. I knew him as a village spokesman, who ran some sort of council. He said, "They have taken our brother and sister. You did not see this, so I must tell you. First they fired a grenade into the house. Then they shot our brother and sister. Then they threw them into the fire and burned the tree. Now there is nothing left."

Another man stepped forward, younger. He had a wild skullcap of curly hair. One of his eyes was jammed inward, staring fixedly at his nose. He said, "It is Ras Hamil who has done this."

I said, "What is your name?"

He said, "I am called Mr. Gugsa."

I looked at the faces of the crowd. The headman looked at Mr. Gugsa, then at me. He nodded. I had come to know a lot of these people over the past five years. Their faces had been shut tight at the beginning. As the hillsides had turned green, the suspicious masks had fallen away. Now the masks were back; the masks of people who remembered what it was like to be hurt, and were not going to let it happen again.

I saw the high, shiny dome of Esias's head in the crowd. I caught his eye. It was heavy with grief and despair. He came toward me, the hem of his robe brushing little plumes from the brown dust. I had a weird, distant feeling: all of this might have been happening to someone else. Esias took my hand, in the way he always took my hand when he had something impor-tant to say. He said, "Now is the beginning of the melting."

I said, "Who is this Ras Hamil?"

At the mention of the name, the eyes slid away. "One of those in the mountains," he said. "Once, a soldier. Now, who knows?" His grip tightened. "Help us," he said. "In the name of your sister, and of God."

I took out a pen and wrote on a piece of paper: *Ras Hamil*. My arms seemed made of chewing gum, stretched until they were ten feet long, remote from my mind.

My nose and mouth were full of the reek of burning. My eyes were blurred with tears. I folded the paper away in the breast pocket of my shirt. Someone using my voice said, "Why?"

The old man who had spoken first said, "It is not for us to know why. We have lost a brother and a sister, each of us. And the tree which was our shade. It is as if we have lost three great trees, not one."

I looked at his earnest black face, the marks of tears above his kinked white beard. I looked at all of them. Saw foreigners whose ignorance had trapped my sister in a place where she had been killed. Beyond them were the rows of closed-up houses and the brown hills, blank as the faces of idiots. I had talked to Esias in his house, but on my terms, not his. I did not understand any of it.

Except that in any dark corner in any little house, any of the millions of little houses in the huge, hot continent, there could be a Kalashnikov, and someone ready to use it.

The size of the place obliterated me. It was vast and cruel, and it did not give a damn. I felt it was ready to squash the white busybody in the crowd by the burned-out tree, the way you squash a mosquito on a wall.

Cold sweat burst on my forehead. My bowels turned to water, and my knees shook. I did not want to stay and find out who had killed my sister and why. I wanted to run away. I pulled the radio out of my pocket. The sweat of fear made it slippery in my hand. I said, "It is safe to land. Get me out of here."

And I waited, shivering with terror, down by the riverbed, while the silver Cessna droned through the wheeling vultures. And I heard Camilla's voice. *You can't not get involved.*

She had got involved.

The Cessna landed. I climbed in. The people of the village

shrank as we climbed away. I stared straight ahead at the murky line of the horizon.

The fear went. Shame flooded in its place. I was the boys' family now. First, I had to tell them.

I was involved, all right.

The horizon blurred and melted.

3

IN ENGLAND I POSTED RHYD'S FINAL BATCH OF TAPES. THE BOYS stayed with me for a sad week, then went back to school. When I had dropped them I drove home to Devon, traveling slowly down the steep-banked lanes on whose sides the primroses were already flowering. At the bottom of the last lane, I turned between two granite obelisks and onto the track that wound down the valley of the River Sweigh to the cottage where Camilla and I had grown up together.

Our father had been vicar of a parish on the outskirts of Kidderminster, an evil Midlands town dedicated to the manufacture of carpets. A small farming grandfather had left him the steep, unproductive river valley, complete with cottage and buildings. Father had used it as a holiday cottage, an antidote to the racket and traffic of Kidderminster. Our mother had died when I was six and Camilla eleven. When our father died eight years later, we had both gone to live in the holiday cottage. It is fair to say that Camilla looked after both my father and me after our mother's death. She was gifted with a great lightness of touch. One of my earliest memories of her was at the age of nine in the gloomy nursery of the red brick vicarage. She had been staging a dolls' tea party. Other little girls bossed their dolls like sergeant majors. Camilla hovered over the table, *persuading* them to do things. It would have been no surprise if they had got up and walked.

We had put ourselves through university. Camilla went to Somerville, where she got her history doctorate at a ridiculously early age and befriended political activists of all hues, many of whom she brought home to the cottage. In another era, she would have disguised herself in men's clothing and gone on crusades. As it was, after college she had worked for a splatter of good causes, ranging from the Pulteney Samaritans to Amnesty International.

Myself, I had the feeling that crusades usually ended in disaster. I had acquired a good degree in zoology and taken to the breeding of endangered species of duck. To Camilla's great amusement and pleasure, I had achieved public recognition for this.

She had met Rhyd when the two of us had been living in the cottage. The light had been blue and soft and Atlantic. The roses had been out, led by the huge, thorny Paul's Himalayan Musk that provided a runway for the rats into the roofspace above the low bedroom ceilings. Camilla had been twenty-six. I had been twenty-one. We had been giggling at the small ads in the *South Hams Gazette*. In those days, Camilla was wearing her blond hair long, so it hung like a yellow curtain on either side of her nose, which was a nice little ski jump to go with the periwinkle blue eyes; California Girl from Devon, with a brand-new doctorate and a will of iron. "Look," she said. "Isn't he *beautiful?*"

She was pointing at the photograph of a man in a cowboy hat. "RHYD WALTERS," said the caption, in Wild West rustic type.

FRIDAY NITE IS COUNTRY NITE AT THE PLYMOUTH HIPPODROME. HEAR HIS HIT SONG "YOU GOT A BEER MAT STUCK TO YOUR FOREHEAD SO I GUESS YOU NEED YOUR SLEEP."

19

The face above the caption had high cheekbones, narrow eyes and a jaw like an outcrop of granite. That evening Camilla went off on her Norton Commando in a tank top, a fringed suede jacket, her tightest Levis, and a pair of Nudie cowboy boots she had picked up in Albuquerque, New Mexico, the summer before. Given the will of iron and the way she looked, it was more or less inevitable that later that night she should have brought back Rhyd Walters on the bike, guitar case and all.

I had been out hauling lobster pots off Danglas Head. When I got back I persuaded myself to go to my office, where the first chapter of the book into which a publisher had persuaded me to expand my dissertation on auks had been sitting for too long. I went out of the house at one in the morning to check that there were no foxes at the cinnamon teal in the pens by the ponds I had dammed into the Sweigh. The sky was crusty with stars. I heard the blare of the Norton, and went back to the house.

Until then I had not classified country singers as human. But Rhyd was different.

He was six foot seven inches tall, with a nasal East Coast voice and hands the size of encyclopedias. He quoted from Virgil in Latin. Camilla's bed was too short for him, so at three o'clock that morning he hauled it down the stairs and out into the garden, where he welded a couple of chunks of angle iron on to the frame. He and Camilla had been visibly in love by breakfast, when I got back from hauling the trammel nets. Rhyd finished his tour, and told Hud Krantz, his manager, that he was unavoidably detained on the wrong side of the Atlantic. Krantz had screamed with rage and horror, because Rhyd had hacked himself a niche in the country music top twenty with his singles, and his albums sold a lot of copies too. Rhyd, as was his wont, had calmed down the opposition, and done exactly as he had intended to do all along. This was to set up in a shed by the Hole, an old victualing dock on the unfashionable swamp at the mouth of the Poult, with a lot of ancient tools he had bought in auctions around Pulteney. In the shed he repaired diesels and anything else mechanical. I helped him when I had time. He wrote a lot of songs for other artists, and played one tour a year to an audience that remained devoted. When he felt the need to express himself in between tours, he played guitar in the Mermaid on Pulteney quay. He converted the barn next to the cottage into a residence for himself and Camilla, and they had got married.

By this time, Camilla was zeroing in on a mission in life. She and Rhyd had had the two boys, Joe and Harry. After a while, Rhyd had got tired of fixing diesels. Meanwhile photographs of the barn were beginning to appear in the kind of magazines whose readers would rather look at pictures of barns than breed. Visitors began trundling down the drive to ask questions about distressed distemper finishes and corn dollies. When Harry was two, I had gone on one of my periodic sailing expeditions, to Spitsbergen to study auks. On my return, Camilla told me that sixty-one perfect strangers had arrived, severally and in groups, to gawp at the renovations to the barn. Both she and Rhyd were developing a hunted, restless look.

One morning, the autumn after that, a white Rolls Royce had picked its way gingerly down the lane, and a stout, hairy man had climbed out. It was October, and I had just brought my nets back from Pulteney Harbor in the pickup. I had them spread on the rough grass of the lawn and was spending a soothing four hours methodically pulling out the desiccated legs of crabs that had got themselves tangled in places where only red mullet had been supposed to be. The stout man wore a shirt unbuttoned to the navel. Gold objects clattered in his chest hair. He looked around him as if he had never seen a net before, or a cottage. He said, in an American accent, "Is this where I find Rhyd Walters?"

I pointed to the barn. He said, "'Preciate that," and waddled gingerly off down the muddy path in his white loafers.

The fat man had turned out to be Hud Krantz, Rhyd's manager and the world's number one country and western impresario. Six weeks later, Rhyd played a spot on Country Cousins, a worldwide TV hook-up concert. The concert raised seven million dollars for famine relief in Africa. New people began visiting the barn: people who would not have recognized a distressed distemper finish if it had socked them on the nose. These people tended to be brown, and thin, and hard talking. A couple of them revealed themselves as surprisingly authoritative about ducks, particularly the domestic breeds of Africa and Southeast Asia. Camilla told me that she and Rhyd had joined PloughShare, a Bristol-based charity stressing appropriate technology, the conversion of military hardware to agricultural uses, and permaculture, whatever that was. I was not greatly interested, because I was in the middle of a long and complicated affair with Mary Morpurgo, who was a poet and had little time for Third World agriculture. Three months after the concert, Camilla and Rhyd put the boys into boarding school in Dorset, climbed onto a plane, and went to live in a village in northern Ethiopia. Soon after they had gone, Mary too had left, telling me that if I thought she was going to spend the rest of her days chasing a lunatic who was fifty percent commando and fifty percent hermit, I was mad. And I had woken up in a world of which they and the boys were no longer a part.

Of course, they had left the barn ready to come back to. But they had never come back.

And now they never would.

I parked the car in the small barn, let myself into the cottage, drank a glass of whiskey and went around the ponds. There had been no foxes. The ducks were all in breeding plumage. I watched the cinnamon teal drake foraging officiously in a muddy corner of his pond while his mate sat patiently on her eggs. Normally I would have been able to sit on a camp stool and freeze what I had seen into a watercolor that would not only identify the duck, but by some process I could not describe give an idea of the way it swam and fed and bred. But as soon as I sat down, I lost sight of the cinnamon teal. My nostrils filled with the bitter smell of ashes, and I was back under the bare black branches of the Alleluia Tree, terrified and ashamed. I folded up the camp stool, went inside, and opened a new bottle.

And that was the way it went for the first two weeks I was back. I tried to paint by day and write poetry by night, and succeeded in doing neither. There was a lot of tidying up to do, the grim kind of tidying up that comes when people have died.

And in the middle of it all, grimmer still, a will arrived from America.

Rhyd must have written it in Ethiopia. He had sent it to his lawyers in somewhere called Quogue, Maine. It was full of the usual legal gibberish, disposing large sums of money in various conventional directions. But there was a peculiar codicil.

What it boiled down to was that he wanted the boys to try living in America, to see if they liked it. In the event of Rhyd and Camilla both dying before the boys were eighteen, they were to spend six months of the year there, under the guardianship of his sister Sarah, of Bethel Bay, Maine. After the first trial period, they could choose to remain either with me or their Aunt Sarah, or to continue as before.

I knew Rhyd had been born on a farm in Maine, into a sect called Christ's Brethren. He had seldom spoken about it or his sister Sarah in my hearing. In the early days, when I had still been worried about what kind of man my sister had handed herself over to, I had looked the Brethren up. Finding nothing in the encyclopedias, I had gone to the London Library, and further.

It had taken two weeks, by the end of which I knew nearly as little as when I had started. All I could dredge up was that in 1682 a John Walters had sailed from Cardiff to the New World, taking with him about sixty men and women whose disgust at the corruption of the established church was so powerful that they had resolved henceforth to consort only with each other. Their ship was called, unsurprisingly, the *Ark*. They had colonized the coast of Maine, and seemed in subsequent years to have dropped almost entirely from the public eye. Their religious observances were characterized by a strong belief in divine inspiration, coupled with an equal belief in divine retribution. They married only among themselves, the few incomers necessary for the vigor of the gene pool being rebaptized and conditioned in an institution known as the Church School. It seemed odd he should want his sons to have anything to do with such people. But he must have discussed it with Camilla, because there it was, stone cold legal, and that was that.

In another codicil he left me his boat, *Halcyon.* I had enough on my mind for now without boats.

I wrote back to the lawyer, saying that the boys would arrive in late spring, the last date permitted. I talked to the boys interminably on the telephone. I organized a memorial service.

It was a good one, if there is such a thing as a good memorial service. We had it in Pulteney Church, which is up on the cliff, crouching behind a windbreak of rhododendrons.

It had been blowing hard all week, proper February gales. The morning of the service, the sun had come out. Outside in the churchyard, daffodils were nodding in the lee of the ramps of boulders propping up the tombstones. To seaward, a big swell was creaming in the rocky fangs of the Teeth. The air across the acid green sea to Danglas Head had the dreamlike transparency that meant it was full of water.

The church was full of people. The boys were out of school for the weekend, looking white and dazed. I had an arm around each of them. Back in the nave, there was most of Pulteney, yachters as well as fishermen; the whole of Plough-Share; Camilla's friends from Somerville and beyond; all the members of the extended family that had made the valley home. The vicar preached, not too long: Greater love hath no man than this, to lay down his life for his friends. I read a poem.

The last hymn was Rhyd's great anthem, the one he had

written for the Country Cousins concert. It had blasted his face all the way around the world. The last verse came around:

> On the final day, the sun rose
> And Lord! then we did see
> There were blood-red flowers blooming
> On the Alleluia Tree.

It broke up the church. We stumbled into the wind that was moaning across a world suddenly blurred and gray. I loaded the boys into the front of the pickup and headed down for the Mermaid on the quay.

The Mermaid had volunteered to clear the pub for our use. The boys went off with Chiefy Barnes to look over the new Arun-class lifeboat delivered a week ago. I drank some whiskey and tried to talk to sympathetic people whose names I had forgotten, and not think about the fact that in my fear I had hurried away from the place Camilla had been killed. Rhyd and Camilla had had a lot of friends. Compared with them, I was more or less a recluse. I did my best with all of them, feeling guilty and miserable, because I had let Camilla down in a big, basic way.

Our father had brought us up to be independent of mind, if not of society. One of my earliest memories was of him sitting in his dark study, the smell of the whiskey he was drinking, the flicker of the black-and-white TV in the corner. On the TV was a march: I suppose it must have been the early 1960s, Ban-the-Bomb. "Silly fools," he said. "Quite right, though."

It took me years to work it out. Making a public fuss, in his view, was a waste of time. Doing private right according to your own conscience was obligatory. Hell was a bad conscience. It went on from there.

Just before he died, I had been watching a goldfinch on the birdtable. I must have said it was beautiful.

"Paint it, then," he said.

I probably said I had never painted anything.

He frowned. His face was gray with the heart disease that killed him. "You've got eyes," he said. "You've got hands."

So I painted it. It never occurred to me to think I might not be able to.

But in the Mermaid, with the people talking solemn talk, I felt a big emptiness. I should have stayed in the village in Ethiopia to find out more. But I had been scared, and had left.

Bad conscience.

I talked to Jerry Stein, the chairman of PloughShare. Jerry was a dynamic individual with white hair and black eyebrows. He was talking about memorial funds; I supposed it was the job of the managers of charities to be alert to methods of turning disasters into money. We were leaning on the bar. So was a large American called Bill something. He said he wanted to talk to me seriously and at length. I did not want to talk to anyone seriously or at length. Shame was riding me like a hag. I gave him my telephone number and went to greet people who needed greeting.

The day after the service, I took the boys back to school. When I came back, the ducks were busy on the ponds and the lawn was covered in the shadows of gulls steadying themselves on the big wind from the sea. It was crowded with animals and ghosts. It was intolerably lonely.

I shoved the ghosts of the valley out of my mind. I went into the workroom, which smelled of paint, and pulled out the folio of preliminary drawings for *North American Ducks*, the book I had promised my editor by April.

It started to rain, a wet thrashing on the big windows. I sat watching the gray curtains drift over the willows that sheltered the duck pens. Down in the valley beyond the willows was the ridge of the barn where Rhyd and Camilla had lived before they had gone to Africa, and been machine-gunned and burned . . .

Pour the last of the bottle into the glass. Drink it. Start again.

Out there beyond the willows and the barn was the sea. It was time to go down to the shed on Pulteney marshes. Touch up *Little Auk*, my ancient yacht. Give her a lick of paint;

overhaul the engine. Maybe another sail, after I had finished the book. Up to the North Cape, paint some birds, walk on some spring flowers. Get alone on the sea and the mountains, without ghosts. Get blown inside out, write some poems, feel alive again.

In previous years, Camilla had helped me paint *Little Auk.*

I shivered. My hand went for the cupboard by the gumboot rack, where the crates lived.

Time for another nice glass of whiskey.

My hand closed on the cool neck of a new bottle.

The telephone rang.

I let it ring. It would be Julia the editor, after *North American Ducks.* Julia was an efficient person who sat in a warm office with schedules on the wall. She was anxious for the next title from George Devis, explorer, sometime paramour of Mary Morpurgo, author and illustrator not only of the respectable *Auks,* but also of the hugely popular *Best Guide to British Birds,* now in its thirteenth edition and showing no signs of flagging. George Devis was about as close as Best Books were ever going to get to the Mother Lode.

I cracked the seal on the new bottle. There were eleven empties in the crate, waiting to go to the bottle bank. Julia always gave up after twelve rings.

It kept right on going after twelve. All right, all right, I thought. I picked it up.

4

*T*HE VOICE ON THE OTHER END WAS AMERICAN, A RAW GROWL THAT sounded as if it might once have played football and now smoked too many cigarettes. "Devis," it said. "I have to see you."

I said, "Who is this?"

"Bill Marsden," he said. "We met at the Mermaid, after the church? I'd like to talk. I just came back from Africa, before the service. I'm someplace called Exeter. How do I reach you?"

I wanted to drink whiskey and pretend to paint ducks, not chat about old and shameful times. I started to tell him I was busy. I did not get a chance.

He said, "This may be inconvenient, but I have eight hours, right? And then I have to go see a guy in Prague."

I found myself giving him directions. An hour later he was on the doorstep: a big man, with a fawn raincoat and a stingy-brim tweed hat, and Devon rain running out of eyebrows like gorse brakes.

"Nice place," he said, still on the doorstep. The willows and the duck enclosures were fading into a murky dusk. He was being polite.

He came in, turning his shoulders sideways to get them through the door. He removed his raincoat with the business-like air of a man who has not much time to do an important bit of work. He was six feet tall, fortyish, with a thick neck and close-cut black hair with a peppering of gray.

"That's Camilla," he said, pulling out a Havana cigar.

His eyes had settled on the composite portrait and self-portrait I had painted of her and me. It had been Camilla's idea. She had been looking at some early duck pictures, of a pair of Mandarins in waterlilies. She said, "Paint us."

I said, "I can't paint portraits."

She said, "How do you know?"

And of course I did not know, so there was nothing more to be said.

In this picture we were sitting on a garden bench, reading the same newspaper. We had lowered the newspaper, looking surprised, who the hell are you? I had too much curly brownish hair, a blurred, beaten-up face, nose broken by a falling volume of the Oxford English Dictionary and skinned by sun on the boat. Camilla was bright blonde, high cheekbones, tough blue eyes. Behind the newspaper we were arm in arm. What remained of the Devis family, ready for anything.

The bitter smell of ashes.

Bill sat down. I said, "So you've been in Africa."

"I was meant to visit with Rhyd and Camilla after you'd left. I went and viewed the . . . ruins."

There was a silence. Outside the window, night was coming down like a wet tarpaulin. I said, "Why?"

He said, "I'm a journalist. I had a professional interest."

"In the land reclamation?"

"Not exactly." He took the cigar out of his teeth. "Rhyd was a kind of versatile guy. He was a good metalworker. He knew a lot about aid, too."

I said, "What are you saying?"

"People can get killed for no reason. I don't think that Rhyd and your sister were like that."

I thought of the slow approach of the olive-drab lorries down the hairpin track from the pass. I thought of the horseshoe of uniformed dolls around the house, the two white faces lifting up their eyes unto the hills, from whence came no help at all. And two hours later, the lorries gone, the naked black limbs of the Alleluia Tree, the pile of ashes. And the ring of black faces, and the waves of terror. I said, "It looked like a military operation." I thought: This man is a reporter. I said, "Have you ever heard of a Ras Hamil?"

The cigar jerked sharply toward me. "Hamil?" he said. "Sure. Why?"

"He killed them."

The dark brown eyes were penetrable as shuttered windows. He said, "How do you know?"

I said, "I was told by . . . eyewitnesses." I could not bear to think about it. It came back anyway.

From the landing strip, Derek had flown me back to the mission. The fear had faded. The grief had taken over. As gently as possible, I told the boys what had happened.

They did not show a lot. I do not think they even understood, not properly. As if you could understand a thing like that, whatever age you were.

We flew to Addis Ababa. I did my best to make a fuss, starting with the British Embassy. The man from the Embassy had shrugged, and said, "Of course there is a problem. This Ras Hamil chap, well, he's a bandit, frightful nationalist, clanking with Russian weapons left over from the civil war, won't talk sense to anyone. Frankly, it's not safe for Europeans up there. I said as much to your brother-in-law." He had popped green eyes, a reddish toothbrush moustache, and a shaving rash. He was not making me feel any better. "Off back home, eh?" he said. "Lucky devil."

I said, "I want to know about Ras Hamil."

His wet red mouth had hung open. He had seemed to have forgotten the name already.

By dint of constant hammering, I had found out whom to bribe. A handful of fivers had landed me in an office in a government building. There was a ceiling fan fluttering the flakes of whitewash that were peeling from the walls. There was a made-in-Russia desk, some years old. Behind the desk was a colonel in a lightweight khaki uniform, eyelids teetering over his sleepy eyes, long black hands looking ready to fall off his wrists.

I said, "The man Ras Hamil has murdered my sister and her husband."

Flies buzzed. The fan rustled the papers on the desk. The colonel said, "This is a very shocking thing."

I said, "What are you going to do about it?"

His long hands moved like waterweeds. "I fear there is very little we can do," he said. "This Hamil is . . . a brigand. You should know that there are great parts of the interior that are temporarily beyond our control. In the hands of emerging democratic groups. Elections will be held, of course. Then we shall see." He did not sound as if he knew what we should see.

I said, "Murder has been committed."

He said, "Alas." He seemed to think he had done enough. There was shouting from outside the window. Someone was battering a drum. He had no more idea where to begin than I had. He was frightened to go into the interior and ask questions. So was I.

He stood up. He said, in his languishing voice, "Allow me to extend my condolences."

The soupy air had flowed away from my face like a ship's bow wave as I left the office. But it was the shame that was making me sweat.

And now the air was cold, and wet, and stank of Havana tobacco. And this Bill was still watching with his dark, empty eyes.

I said, "So what do you know about Ras Hamil?"

"Warlord," he said. "Sorry. Leader of emerging democratic political grouping." The Ethiopian colonel had used the same slab of jargon. "Come out of nowhere. Just beginning to put himself about a little. Nobody knows anything about him. Runs a semiprivate army of about ten thousand guys. Will shortly be running for election, if they get around to having elections. You talk to the guys in Addis, he frightens the hell out of them."

I said, "How is killing Rhyd and Camilla a good electoral move?"

He disappeared for a moment behind a blue gray veil of smoke. He said, "That is what I was asking the people in the village. I guess some people would tell you that Rhyd and Camilla were patronizing neocolonialist power freaks."

"Not the people in the village."

He said, "By the time I got there, there were two corn dealers selling stuff. And there were a couple of people who said they were Baptist missionaries, but you can't ever tell. There wasn't any Rhyd or Camilla to tell them to go to hell. So the corn dealers were after the spare cash, and I guess the missionaries are either missionaries or they want to start some kind of cash crop they can buy cheap, truck out of there and sell. I don't know. All I know is that when Rhyd was around the people in the village would talk to you, and now he isn't around they won't talk to anybody any more, because they have been shown that the Rhyd and Camilla method gets you shot and burned." He flicked ash off the cigar. "So they were real scared. And they didn't tell me anything."

I thought of the closed-up faces after the burning. We had all been scared, but I had had an exit. I said, "Why were you asking the questions?"

He said, "It's my job. I'm a reporter. Boston *Echo.* I guess you won't have heard of it."

I had not. I said, "You were a long way from home."

He said, "I have a . . . special interest in the story." His face was suddenly not the impenetrable face of someone whose job it is to ask questions. There was a softening about the mouth and eyes and he looked at the whiskey in his glass as if he wanted to avoid looking at anything else. "Rhyd was an old friend," he said. "We had an argument before he came over here to live with your sister. I told him he was crazy. So he explained. He said that country music was no occupation for a grown-up human being, and that your sister had shown him how grown-up human beings behave. We talked about that." He laughed. "I'm a reporter, right? Professional skeptic. I don't believe in anything but the story. But I believed in Rhyd and Camilla, all right." He reached for the whiskey bottle. "So that's why I'm here."

I watched the slight tremor of his hand as he poured a slug. The lamplight gleamed on his forehead, as if the admission had cost him effort. I said, "I don't understand."

"I'm sorry," he said. "I'm not expressing myself too well. What I mean is, you and I are kind of in a similar relation to Rhyd and Camilla. Closely peripheral, you could say. So I didn't like what I saw in that village. I'd like to raise the funds to get somebody else out there to carry on the work. Yes?"

I thought of Camilla. I thought of the fear, and the way I had let her down. What Bill was saying might help. I said, "Of course."

He was back on track now, his eyes sharp as needles under the heavy eyebrows. He had a poker player's face, full of cleverness. He said, "I have a plan."

I did not say anything. He had a confident presence, this Bill.

"Rhyd said you're a sailor." He grinned. "Actually, he said you had done some real extreme things in a real old boat. I read your book about Spitsbergen. You sailed up there by yourself?"

Put that way, it sounded brave and splendid. The truth had been less dramatic.

I had been writing the dissertation on auks as part of my degree. The way I saw it, there were two choices. One was to sit in a library with occasional side trips to the coastal waters of Europe for field study. The other was to visit Spitsbergen, auk capital of the world, for which I had no prospect of raising fares or visas.

I had just broken up with a girlfriend whose craving for a social life was stronger than mine. Furthermore I had *Thug*, a boat that I had resurrected from a scrapyard when I was sixteen and rebuilt with the help of some friends in Pulteney, Charlie Agutter among them. It was what would now be called a classic. It was immensely solid, twenty-eight feet long, built of oak planks on oak frames. So I provisioned this boat and, without telling anyone (in case they managed to persuade me not to go), I started north. I touched the Shetlands, Tromsö and Spitsbergen, then an armed camp across which NATO and the Soviets were glaring at each other. I saw seven million auks. Thanks to insane luck with the weather and the navigation, I failed to drown. When I came home, I found myself mildly notorious. I turned the dissertation into a book and an Anglia wildlife film. Camilla had pretended to find the whole business hilarious, but I knew she was proud as hell.

So the Spitsbergen trip had served its purpose: no more, no less.

I said, "I haven't done that kind of thing for a long time."

There was a silence. Rain rattled on the windows. Then he said, suddenly, "I brought back Rhyd's ashes."

"His *what?*"

"His ashes. I want to take them home. I'm going to take the urn to his sister Maria, in conditions of maximum publicity."

I stared at him. "Maria?"

"Wait," he said. "I intend to secure maximum publicity by sailing them across the Atlantic in a boat. I intend to sail this boat in the Weston's Two-Handed Early Atlantic Race. Starts in a month. Boat's name will be changed to *PloughShare*. Lecture tour arranged in New England, Rhyd's home ground, household goddamn name, talk to ladies who lunch, donations invited. I know how to do that. You can speak in public, I have heard. We'll clean up."

I said again, "Maria?"

"Rhyd's sister."

"You found her?"

He frowned at me. "Sure," he said. "Or she found me."

"Rhyd hadn't seen her for years. He didn't know where she was."

"She wouldn't tell him where she was. She contacted me when she heard he was dead. Rhyd's family are . . . kind of weird. He talk to you about them?"

"Hardly at all."

"I guess Maria couldn't take the pressure they handed out. You know?"

The only clue about the pressure had been Rhyd's refusal to talk about them. I said, "So this race. Have you got a boat?"

He said, "No. But you do. Do you want to go with me?"

I sat there and listened to my heart. It was beating heavily, like a muffled drum. I had known him for a total of forty minutes, and he wanted to sail across the Atlantic.

His eyes were like Billy Graham's. Take-up-thy-bed-and-walk eyes. Like Camilla's. He said, "Rhyd was telling me, letter he wrote one time, that you are a real fussy bastard and you keep that boat in real good shape. I already spoke to the committee. They prequalified us, in view of your past record. Hell, so we come last. I'll scare up a lot of press the other end. There'll be a lecture tour. We'll raise a lot of money."

I said, "Wait a minute."

He relit his cigar, which had gone out. He fixed me with the Billy Graham eyes. He said, "Maybe just another taste of that excellent whiskey?"

I threw a couple of logs into the stove. It was dark outside. Bill allowed the eyes to rest on the portrait of me and Camilla. He said, "That picture by you? It's good." He drank. "It fries my ass. I was only a friend. She was your sister. There's no comparison. How are the kids?"

I said, "It's early to tell." The boys were due at their Aunt Sarah's in America in May, after half-term. The race would give me an excuse for being there when they arrived. It would not be impossible to arrange.

Bill blew smoke, refilled his glass. He said, "How are you feeling?"

I had not even talked to myself about how I was feeling. I thought: Here is some bastard who barges in here full of romantic bloody notions of memorial transatlantic lecture tours, drinks your whiskey, smokes cigars all over your studio. There is no need to confide in him. I looked at the portrait of Camilla. I thought of the green bowl in the dun hills, the hoarse voices in the workshop. Into the emptiness came her voice. *You can't not get involved.* A lecture tour could raise funds to reestablish the project in the village. Buy off a few tons of the shame.

I said, "Why are you doing this?"

Bill said, "You have to remember your friends."

I thought about that. My problem was that I remembered them too intensely. I told myself that what I wanted was to forget.

But what I was trying to forget was not Rhyd or Camilla. It was the things Camilla had said to me, the last night of her life. *Tell people what you've seen.* Shortly after which I had run away before I had looked properly.

I said, "And there's a story in it for you."

He shrugged. He said, "We have to eat. I'm owed a month's vacation. I can stretch that. And we can use the paper to give some publicity to the lecture tour. Rhyd was real popular in New England. We'll use that. And we can do some straight talking to the serious money." He delved into his briefcase and came out with a piece of paper. "I did some groundwork," he said.

On the paper were a dozen names and addresses in New England. None of them meant anything to me. "Lunch dates," he said. "We get the far end, make some noise about ashes, give lectures about PloughShare. We'll send 'em a million dollars. Think: What could Rhyd and your sister have done with a million dollars?"

He was grinning. I found I was grinning back. I said, "And then you go back to work."

"Like I said," he said. "I have some vacation owing. Can you think of anything better to do with it?"

I looked out of the window at the garden. There was a bower out there with a Pink Perpetual rose scrambling over it. Rain was dripping from the thorns and on to the stone seat below. The stone seat had been the center of activities in the summers before Rhyd had arrived. I had found it in a junkyard and carved a new wing for the gryphon that supported the right-hand end of the seat.

It was on the stone seat that I had been sitting with Mary Morpurgo one day in July, a couple of years after the Spitsbergen trip. Morpurgo was someone Camilla had met in a drinking club in Soho and brought home because she thought she was interesting and in need of a holiday. She had curly black hair and green eyes and a bony Celtic nose. At that precise moment she was wearing only a pair of bikini bottoms. There was a dragon tattooed on the nut-brown skin of her right shoulder, and a wreath of briony on her right ankle. Mary was the author of five books of poetry, and was as famous as a poet could be in England. She was also a practicing witch. Just then, she was stroking her right breast, the nipple of which was standing out like a brown thimble. I was watching this with great interest; Mary's body was as dramatic as her mind. She was also expounding her theory that everyone was a poet.

"Mmm," she said after a while, edging along the bench and leaning against me. "I wonder, could you come and do this for me?"

The talk about poetry then ceased. But when I could think again I thought about what she had said. I had no idea how you started writing poetry. So I took my school Virgil out of the big bookcase on the cottage stairs and translated the first eclogue into a sort of verse. I found it the same sort of problem as a painting, only harder. Mary had stayed on. She told me she liked the translation; but Mary liked everything about me then, the way I liked everything about her.

I wrote more poems, including (a year later) the New Eclogues, pastoral poems for a world on the edge of chaos. People took a lot of notice of it, and Mary—who by then was living in the cottage—had persuaded me to go on a reading tour with her.

So I had begun performing in public. I did not mind the performances; after all, if you had written something, you might as well make sure people read it the way it was intended. What I objected to were the frauds who clung to the poets;

bureaucrats on one end, people with shaved heads and velvet hats on the other. Mary loved them, because they sat still for her earth magics in community-center dressing rooms in Telford. After five tours, it got to the point where I was going to say something that would make everybody very cross, and change nothing. So I left the tour, and entered the Round the Islands Race with my childhood friend Charlie Agutter in *Auk*, the boat I had bought with the proceeds of the *Best Book of British Birds*.

Sail across the Atlantic with this Bill. A bit of public speaking.

Blot out the shame.

No problem.

I picked up the telephone, dialed the number of Charlie Agutter. He was a yacht designer as well as a childhood friend. He was in charge of the structural health of *Little Auk*.

I said, "How long would it take to get *Auk* ready for a transatlantic?"

"I was down there today," he said. "She's very tidy. Full blast, two weeks."

I thought for a moment, while the whiskey rang in my ears. "Right," said a voice, "let's do it." It was my own voice. "I'll be down in the morning."

"Bring some lists," said Charlie. *"Hasta luego."*

I put the telephone down. I said, "I hope you do not regret this."

"I won't," said Bill, and grinned all the way around his cigar.

What I meant was that I hoped I would not regret it.

Next morning at ten I rang Eddie Floyd at *The Yachtsman*. He sobered up enough to tell me that Bill had been unnecessarily modest when he told me he had done a transatlantic. He had also sailed a singlehanded Bermuda race and written a book about cruising the Pacific. On the whole, Eddie thought, there would be very little difficulty.

I rang up Julia, the editor, told her that *North American Ducks* would have to wait, and slammed the telephone down on her

CLAWHAMMER

pleas for mercy. I then rang the boys' headmaster, the race organizers, and Jerry Stein at PloughShare. After that I went down to the yard and started work.

When Rhyd had told Bill I was a fussy bastard about *Little Auk*, he had not been far from the truth. Most of the royalties from the *Best Book of British Birds* went into her upkeep. She was an old-style ocean racer, built in 1937, one of the first yachts to carry a masthead rig. In her day, she had sailed the competition under the water. Now she was an old lady, but tough with it. She had been refastened the previous year. Charlie Agutter knew a couple of shipwrights down at the Hole, and Bill Tyrrell, the local big-old-boat proprietor, gave me a lot of help based on his experience with his antique cutter *Vixen*. So we renewed the standing and running rigging, found a reconditioned generator to attach to *Auk*'s none-too-brilliant wiring, and painted the name *PloughShare* on everything in sight. After a fortnight of this, I discovered to my surprise that I had not yet drunk the remaining half of the twelfth bottle of whiskey.

Bill went to Prague, returned, and joined in the work. I watched him closely, the way you will watch a complete stranger on whom your life is going to depend. He overhauled *Auk*'s engine, a Perkins 4.107 of great age and suspect reliability. As we went over the boat together he worked hard and consistently, twenty hours a day, never asking to be passed a tool or losing his sense of humor.

By the third week, we had spent a lot of time in each other's society. I knew I could rely on him to sail a boat, maintain a boat, and look after himself. I knew he was unmarried and was a senior reporter on the Boston *Echo*. I knew he took size eleven sea boots. And I knew he was committed to raising money for PloughShare.

But that was all. In the circumstances, it seemed enough.

So a week before the race, we sailed around to Plymouth. We were based in the Queen Anne's Battery marina, on the eastern side of the harbor. *Auk* (I could not get used to calling her *PloughShare*) lay rafted up with big plastic multihulls and state-of-the-art sixty-foot monohulls painted candy colors.

With her white hull and wooden spars she had the air of a maiden aunt at a roller disco.

At eight o'clock on the morning of the twenty-first day after Bill's arrival on the doorstep, the big orange-and-blue Pulteney lifeboat appeared around the breakwater. I had a dry mouth, partly because of the two parties I had been to the previous night, and partly because in three hours the race began.

There were a lot of people on the lifeboat's bow. Charlie Agutter was there with two smaller figures alongside. The three of them jumped off the lifeboat and on to the breakwater, then clambered across the raft of boats on to *Little Auk*'s deck.

Charlie said, "Brought these guys down for the day."

Charlie was a brilliant helmsman as well as an internationally famous yacht designer. He was also a very kind man. He still pulled lobster pots, and in the days of the old Pulteney lifeboat had been a regular crew member. The boys thought he was God.

Joe and Harry were out of uniform, grinning like chimpanzees. Joe said, "You've got the boat looking nice."

Harry said, "Is that the salt horse I hear neighing?"

We sat in the cockpit. There was nothing left to do, so we drank tea and talked for twenty minutes. People around us were unrafting. I said to Joe and Harry, "Haul down the battle flag."

They went forward, cocky under the eyes of the spectators on the breakwater, hauled the green flag with the gold plough down from the forestay and brought it aft.

Harry handed me the flag, bowing a deep and courtly bow. To someone who knew him as well as I did, he was looking nervous. He and his brother had been left alone in the world once already this year.

He said, "Did you know you're famous?" He pulled a folded sheet of newspaper out of the back pocket of his jeans and opened it out.

There was a picture of Bill and me at a party on someone's boat. Bill looked big and shambling, grinning amiably. I was a head shorter, looking narrowly at the camera like a middleweight boxer in need of a haircut. I do not like having my photograph taken. Mary Morpurgo used to say I was worried about someone stealing my soul, but then that was the sort of thing Mary said. The caption said "PULTENEY MAN HEADS WEST ON SAD ERRAND." The story spoke of sponsorship and ashes.

"You look a right thug," said Joe. He had a copy of the paper, too.

"Hey!" said Bill. "Can I have that, when you're all done?"

Harry looked at me. So did Joe. I saw that they wanted the papers as souvenirs; souvenirs not only of the race, but of their uncle, their only link with life as it had been before it had been torn up by the roots. I said, "Bill, you can buy your own. Why don't you autograph your photo and shut up?"

Bill looked between us. He saw, and understood, and was embarrassed. He grinned and went below.

Joe said, "Well. See you in America."

Harry said, "Best of British luck, old fruit."

I said, "I'll ring the headmaster. You can follow us on Argos."

Harry said, "What?"

Joe said, "It's a satellite tracking system." He pointed at the blister aerial on the back end of the boat. "Keeps the race committee up to date."

Trust Joe to know.

The lifeboat nosed around the corner. They hopped aboard. We cast off. They stood there waving as we passed out into the big blue harbor and headed for the gap in the breakwater.

The lifeboat hovered out there, clear of the sixty-one competitors. The multihulls roared to and fro dragging plumes of spray like waterskiers, their helmsmen posing for the TV cameras in the helicopters. On the gun, they put their noses across the westerly breeze and vanished in the general direction of Spain. Bill and I waved to the lifeboat, drank a glass of whiskey and played Jimi Hendrix's *Star-Spangled Banner* on the new stereo presented to us by Fore Street Audio of Pulteney. *Auk* tucked her shoulder in and began to bob and plunge south.

The lifeboat shrank astern. It pulled a toot on its siren,

turned 180 degrees and headed back for Pulteney, shrinking on the blue and sparkling sea.

I took a swig of whiskey and turned my mind away from home. Now we were at it, the old excitement was returning. The wind backed southerly. We proceeded for the Lizard and Scilly, and thence on to a Great Circle course for Newport, Rhode Island.

5

*T*HIRTY-SIX DAYS LATER, I WOKE UP EXHAUSTED AT EIGHT P.M., and everything was as usual. Opposite my aching eyes was a bunk; uphill, but not far enough uphill to mean that there was any breeze to speak of. Above the bunk was the shelf of books. Above the shelf was the line of round gray portholes.

On a good day, the portholes were little blue discs of sky. On a bad day, they were gray.

I sat up. My body moaned that three hours' sleep was not enough. The air in the cabin felt cold and dank, full of the fog sliding in a slow gray blanket over the shallow Eastern Atlantic. We had been sliding ourselves, in the boat, blue at first, then fog gray. We had only a dead reckoning plot to tell us where we had slid to, because the batteries and the alternator had been out for a week, and the standby generator's impressive electronic ignition was dead as mutton, and there had been no sun or stars for the sextant, and the Argos satellite position indicator on the transom was for the use of the race committee and commentators, not us. When the radio had last worked, our position in the race had been last.

What we needed was a really good electrical repair shop, closely followed by a hot shower. There are very few of these a hundred-odd miles south of Cape Sable. Besides which, when the crew of the boat consists only of George Devis and Bill Marsden, both of them in the last stages of sleep deprivation, there is very little time for mending anything.

So out there it was gray, and cold, and foggy. The boat was more or less broken, and I had no idea where we were. It was the kind of thing you got used to, sailing *Little Auk*. It was the kind of thing that had made Camilla laugh, and seriously irritated Mary Morpurgo.

I rolled my legs out of the sleeping bag and straight into my boots. I stood up, groaned, pumped water into the kettle, pushed on the whistle and slapped it on to the stove. I lit the gas, dived into my coat, and gave the barometer a sharp, ill-tempered rap. It was a cute barometer, old-fashioned, like *Little Auk*. Sorry, *PloughShare*.

I pulled up the zip on the coat and slid back the hatch.

Bill was standing at the tiller, hands in pockets, football player's shoulders hulking against the pearl-gray sky at his back. I said, "Tea coming."

He said, "Terrific." He looked to his left, into the mist. "Company."

I clambered up the companionway and stepped into the cockpit. *Little Auk*'s deck stretched away forward: cabin top, mast, foredeck, big foresail. We were moving very slowly, about the speed of a gull swimming, across an oily swell as gray as the sky.

The fog was coming and going. One moment there was no forestay. The next, a bank of the stuff had slid back and we were drifting across the silky floor of a crater of brownish-gray vapor.

"There," said Bill.

I had got it.

Stuck in one of the fogbanks like a mammoth in an iceberg was a low, dark hull with a squat funnel, upperworks and what looked like derricks on its afterdeck. "Fishing boat," I said.

"Scallop dragger," he said.

"Has he seen us?"

Bill shrugged. Normally he would have been below by now, groping his way into his sleeping bag for his four hours off. But a fishing boat meant a lot of things, all of them worth staying awake for. For one thing, *Little Auk* was only thirty-eight feet long, with a small radar signature. A fishing boat could go straight through her and feel as little as a lorry crossing a pothole.

For another, the little windows on the shiny new plastic boxes above *Auk*'s chart table had been blank since the electrics had gone. Fishing boats had plastic boxes of their own. We could check our dead reckoning. I pulled the foghorn out of its clips and blew. The sound rolled across the water like the blare of a bull.

The fishing boat was turning from beam-on to end-on, the mast moving in line with the funnel. Bill was waving now, tiller gripped between his knees.

We were a couple of hundred yards apart and closing. I went below and pulled *Auk*'s old brass megaphone out of the net locker aft of the chart table. Bill said, "Gimme the grab bag." The kettle started to whistle. I passed the grab bag up through the hatch, turned off the gas, made the tea. As I turned back to the companionway, Bill had his Nikon up to his eye, taking a photograph of the fishing boat. I ran up the companionway. He put the camera back in the grab bag. The fishing boat had turned beam-on again, a hundred and fifty feet across the water. Her side was tar-black with a deep rubbing strake. We were close enough to see the scratches and gouges. There was a number under the bow. I raised the megaphone to my mouth. I shouted, *"What is our position?"*

"He can't hear you," said Bill.

A man came out of the fishing boat's wheelhouse. He was

wearing a black oilskin that gleamed faintly in the fog. The boat looked solid and competent; there were aerials on her wheelhouse, and her derricks clanked in the swell. Friendly. In touch with the world. The first humans we had seen for the best part of a month.

Bill said, "Give that to me."

I handed him the megaphone. My throat was dry, my mouth gluey. I had not had the cup of tea yet. Bill put the megaphone to his mouth. The man on the fishing boat's deck raised something. Loudhailer, I thought.

It was not a loudhailer.

Against the dark loom of his shoulder came into being a little jumping flame. With the flame, keeping time, there came a hard clatter like a riveting gun. Metal clanged on metal. The megaphone spun away. It was an old megaphone, part of the boat. I liked the megaphone. I was half asleep. I opened my mouth to shout.

Bill said, *"Oof."*

I stared at him. My mouth was still open, but the shout had not arrived. My mind was on freeze frame. My heart had stopped beating.

He looked at me with surprised eyes. He said, "Bag label." Blood started running from his mouth and down his chin.

I fell flat on my face in the bottom of the cockpit, looking up. I could see Bill's head and shoulders against the fog. I yelled, "Down!"

The riveting gun started again.

Bill's head blew off.

He stood there in the fog, his shoulders big as ever. But the line of the shoulders continued straight across. There was no neck. Something made a heavy plunging sound in the sea alongside.

I looked at him with my mouth still open.

In the gray fog, a red rain began. Beyond the rain, I heard engines roar. Little stinging things flew through the air. Bill's body lurched away from the tiller and slammed on to the deck. Glass was breaking.

Machine gun, I thought, with a mind that might have belonged to a stranger. All your life you are nowhere near machine guns. Then you are right there, twice in four months.

The engines roared, came closer. I stayed down, groveling on the slippery red deck. There was fog inside my head as well as out. *Auk* began to heel, heading up into the wind. The machine gun stopped. The noise of engines came closer. I might have been crying.

There was a heavy crash. The deck smacked me in the ear, heeled steeply; Bill's blood ran in a red lake across the cockpit. His body rolled off me. I saw the scarred black side of the fishing boat slide by six feet away. He had rammed us. I kept dead still. I was very frightened.

The engine clattered again. There was the roar of water on a rudder. The deck heaved. The air smelled of fog, and blood, and old fish. The fishing boat was very close, pulling his nose out of *Auk's* side.

He came back in.

This time, his bow hit *Auk* amidships. The sound was more a crunch than a crash. *Auk* began to slew sideways, the fisherman's bow buried in her flank. I lay rigid, too scared to move, watching the blank gray reflections in the wheelhouse windows thirty feet away. I could feel something sticky on my face. Blood. Wind roared in *Auk's* sails and tormented wood set up a complaining squeal down in her bowels. Something said *snap*. Shroud, I thought. The mast came down, slowly, like a tree. It was a tall mast, forty-five feet long. It came down on the fishing boat's wheelhouse, sail and all. More glass broke. I heard American swearing. Bill, I thought. Then I realized that it was coming from the wheelhouse, which had vanished under the sail.

And Bill had no head.

I moved.

There was a life raft stowed on the back end of the cockpit. I tossed it overboard. I was shaking so much I could hardly walk the two steps. I pulled the quick release and the life raft hissed, swelled into a yellow doughnut with a roof. The fishing boat's engine was hammering. Quick, I thought. Quick. Bill's body was only a thing. The grab bag. I stooped, grabbed the bag, tumbled over the stern and into the life raft, let go the painter. For a moment I saw the fishing boat, its high, gray axe of bow sunk in *Little Auk*'s side. *Little Auk* heeled steeply, her sail smothering the wheelhouse. The fishing boat throttled up, ploughed on, shoving *Little Auk* across the water at perhaps five knots. A smooth gray swell came between me and it. The mast had come upright and rolled away from the fishing boat. Next time I could see, the fog was thickening again. There was a grinding of steel on timber; a huge, flatulent thunder of bubbles. The fog came down. *Auk* and Bill were gone.

Five minutes ago I had rolled out of my bunk and put the kettle on. Now I was floating in a rubber dinghy in a finger of the Labrador current, with an emergency supply pack and a camera bag half-full of blood.

I had not even had a cup of tea.

I hung my head over the side, and shook, and was sick.

The fog was thick as porridge. I could hear engines out there. The seas boomed and throbbed in the grayout. Wash cut across the swell, making the dinghy lurch and roll. I lay in the bottom and prayed for the fog to be thicker, the dusk sooner, the current bigger. And I prayed in a most primitive and infantile manner that I would live.

There was a surge of wake, a heavy whiff of diesel in the gray nothing. Engines rumbled in my bones, faded away. I was left in the cold gray silence. Alone, somewhere in the Atlantic.

Alone was fine. The shaking would not stop. Busy, busy, I thought. Keep the circulation going. Water temperature maybe forty degrees, a couple of thicknesses of rubberized fabric away. My surroundings were a little orange-and-gray hut on a rubber ring the size of a tractor inner tube.

I tore open the emergency kit and got tremendously practical. Work, don't think.

First there was the EPIRB—Emergency Position Indicating Radio Beacon—like an orange flashlight with an aerial. I twisted the plastic base. The red light came on and radio waves began pulsing on the distress frequency, notifying airliners and satellites that someone was in bad trouble somewhere down here in the fog south of Cape Sable. The Argos signal on the boat would have gone out, too. There would be alarms blinking. The boys would worry. No thinking allowed, though. A man could go crazy, thinking. I had a little cookery session, featuring a rip-top foil bag of fresh water and a glucose tablet. This was not technically demanding, but it seemed to take forever, because my hands felt as if I was wearing boxing gloves, and I was seeing the world through many thicknesses of none-too-clean polythene. Shock, said the family doctor who lives back in the head. General shutdown in the face of overload.

So most of the glucose and water went down the outside of my neck. And I lay there, and saw once again the line of Bill's shoulders running straight across, no neck, and felt the hot red rain, and heard that big, horrible plunging noise. It made me think of another rain, the belch of black smoke jumping into the blue African sky from the bungalow. It seemed to be night, which of course was wrong. Around the bungalow, a circle of men in green uniforms poured white tracers on to the red fire. The Cessna with only me in it, scared stomachless, turned away from the horrible bonfire. The bonfire became a sunset, and the sunset shrank into an orange pinpoint, to be swallowed up in the enormous, terrifying blackness of the African night.

Except that it was not hot enough for Africa, and not black enough. It was a cold, gray world, and a small one. It turned colder, and grayer, and I think I did a lot of yelling.

Finally, after a very long time, there was noise.

At first I thought it was the fishing boat. But it came from above: a hellish *whock* of rotors and the roar of an engine. And a voice was saying something I could not hear above the racket. I did not listen much. I was saying, "Bag." The grab bag was important. I scrabbled for it, put the strap around my neck. The roof of the life raft opened like an egg hatching and let in a white hot glare of searchlights from above. A visored helmet bore the words U.S. COAST GUARD. A loop of webbing tightened under my arms. We ascended into a new world.

Me and the grab bag.

6

I WOKE UP IN A COOL WHITE ROOM. OUTSIDE THE PLATE-GLASS
window, white clouds were sailing across a sky of rainwashed
blue. The room smelled of hospitals, but the disinfectant was
wrong. I wondered why. A button by my bed said NURSE. A
pretty blond girl in uniform came in. She said, "Hi there!" Her
accent was American, of course, and she had spectacular teeth.
For the first time in my life, I was in the United States of
America.

She said, "How are you doing?"

Talking was like pushing a big car uphill. I said, "I had a
bag."

She ignored me. She said, "We have Dr. Finestone outside,
okay? And there are some other folks."

I said, "The bag."

She left, still ignoring me.

With a huge effort, I got myself up on to a pile of pillows. It
was surprisingly difficult. The doctor came in. He told me I had
shock, and hypothermia, and showed me a kidney bowl of
wood splinters he had pulled out of various parts of me. I

looked at the pile of little brown needles, and thought for a moment about *Little Auk* and the summers I had spent keeping her afloat, brushing out varnish on her brightwork and recaulking her vile old decks so Mary Morpurgo could stretch her tattooed body thereupon.

Then I said, through a mouthful of marbles, "Where is this?"

The doctor smiled. His teeth were almost as white as the nurse's. "Portland, Maine," he said. "George Morrow Hospital."

The fog in my mind lifted an inch or two. Top righthand corner of America, I thought. By the sea. Just below where the coast starts to get ragged and Norwegian looking.

The doctor said, *"PloughShare* was the boat. You're George?"

The map vanished. The fog thickened. I said, "How did you guess?"

"Name was on your life raft. The race people reported you missing when your Argos went out." He was brown haired, tanned. He looked fit, and he wore Docksiders under his white coat. "Someone run you down?"

I said, "Where's my bag?"

"Customs and Immigration are waiting to meet with you. Your bag's with them. They won't give you any trouble."

I said, "How long have I been here?"

"Thirty-six hours. You've been shocked real bad. We want to hold you under observation for four or five days."

I said, "Is that compulsory?"

The doctor grinned. His grin was as white as the nurse's. Bill was dead. The grin was meant to tell me: Life goes on. "This is the Land of the Free," he said. "But if we let you out early, you might sue."

He was fading. My eyes were heavy. I did not mind how long I stayed in this soft bed with the clouds sailing by outside the window. I went to sleep.

Next time I woke, a nurse brought me what she said was a Salisbury steak, which turned out to be some kind of hamburger with mashed potato, and a cup of coffee. I gave her the number of the boys' school and asked her to call the headmaster and tell the boys I was fine. Then she showed in a gray-haired man in uniform. He said, "Good afternoon," eased the gun in the holster on his right buttock, and sat down in a low chair. I chewed wearily on some mashed potato and asked him what day it was. He said, "Monday, sir. I have to take a statement."

So I told him what had happened. He wrote it down slowly in a notebook. When I had finished, he said, "So you didn't see a name on this dragger?"

"No name," I said. "Can't remember."

"No," he said. "Well, thank you, Mr. Devis. That was a real scientific statement. Er . . . can you think of anyone who could want you dead?" He said *day-ud.* The word brought back the straight, headless line of Bill's shoulders. I closed my eyes. The crowd in Ethiopia was waiting for me in the dark, and the fear, and the shame.

I opened my eyes again. I said, "Not unless someone wanted to make sure he knocked us out of last place in the race." The policeman was staring at me. "Joke," I said.

"Sure." His big slab of a face looked as if he thought I was mad. I could not be sure he was wrong. "You say you asked this dragger for your position. I guess maybe that wasn't so tactful."

I said, "What do you mean?"

He said, patiently, as if to a child, "People here in the United States consume a whole heap of narcotics. Plenty of it comes in from the sea. So my bet would be that you asked some guy carrying dope where you were, and he felt his life would be simpler if you folks had an accident."

I said, "He tried to kill two people. In cold blood." Cold was not the word. I felt the hot rain in the gray fog. My gorge rose. The policeman and the clouds outside the window started to flicker.

He said, "If those guys had a couple million dollars' worth of coke in the fish bins, I guess they would have wanted to be real discreet." He stood up. "We'll do our best, but I don't hold out a whole lot of hope. Well, I'll be on my way. Man outside wants to talk about your bag."

A picture flashed across my inner eye. Bill standing in the cockpit with the Nikon, and his head. My stomach did a backflip. I said, with difficulty, "There's a camera in the bag. It's got a photograph of the boat in it. On it." My mind was slipping gears.

The policeman looked mildly enthusiastic. "Zat right?" he said. "I might borrow that for a while, okay?"

I said it was okay. He got me to sign a receipt with a pen that seemed excessively heavy. Then he left.

Another man came in; smaller, olive-skinned, in a different uniform. He sat on the hard chair. On the Formica table beside him he put a blue waterproof camera bag. He ran his hand over his black moustache, and said, "Is this your bag, Mr. Devis?"

I said, "It is the ship's grab bag, so I know what's in it."

He said, "How's that?"

I said, "It's got everything you want to take with you in an emergency." Except a machine gun, I thought. "In that bag there was a Nikon camera, which I expect the police have taken. You will also find a box of Romeo y Julieta cigars, half full. There are our passports, our wallets, the boat's papers. And an urn."

"An urn?" said the customs man.

"A bronze urn," I said. "Sealed. It contains the ashes of my brother-in-law, Rhydian Walters. Maybe you listen to country and western music?"

"Sure do," said the customs man. "Rhyd Walters? Like, 'The Alleluia Tree'?"

"That's right," I said.

"I heard he died," said the customs man. "I'm not a real big country fan, but . . . well. Holy shit," he said. "Rhyd Walters, huh?" He opened the bag, pulled out the urn, held it reverently in his hands and wagged his head from side to side. "Holy *shit*," he said.

I was getting tired of the fan club. I cleared my throat.

He came to, put the urn on the bedside table and did things in my passport with stamps and staplers. "Er . . . welcome to the United States of America, Mr. Devis."

He left. I rolled my head sideways on the pillow and looked at the urn.

It was a small urn, greenish, with a luggage label tied to what an antique dealer would have called a knop or finial on the lid, as if someone might one day want to take the top off. It was hard to imagine why anyone would want to take the top off. What was inside was presumably about a pint of ashes.

Rhyd and Camilla would not have been interested in ashes. Nor, just now, was I.

I dozed my way through some darkness and some light. When I woke again, my arms felt less like lengths of wool, and the blond nurse seemed less overpowering. She said, "I was real sorry to hear about what happened."

It was hard not to smile. It was good to be sympathized with, particularly by someone with nice big eyes. But the doctor came in again, and she stood to attention while he looked me over. He said, "I guess you're about ready to face the press. You want I should throw 'em in?"

The press was why I was here. I had obligations to Rhyd and Camilla and PloughShare. And now to Bill. I said, "Sure."

There were only four of them. One of them was from the Portland *Intelligencer,* two were from a TV station I had never heard of, and one was from *Yachts,* a sailing magazine. They all asked what had happened, and I told them. Then they wanted to know about my home town, and the boat, and my views about America and drug dealers.

I did not want to talk about any of this. I collected some reserves of energy and said, "The real story here is this. The boat I was sailing was called *PloughShare.* PloughShare is a charity. Rhyd Walters, who was married to my sister, was murdered while he was working for PloughShare. We were bringing his ashes home. This was both a memorial and a fund-raising trip."

They smiled, the skin-deep smile of reporters who know better than you the slant they are going to inflict on their readers. "That the country singer?" said the man from *Yachts.* "Sure," I said. "You've heard of him?"

"I guess most everybody has." He had a jowly, suntanned face with a big moustache and a synthetic fleece pullover. He was frowning. "My readers don't pay a whole lot of attention to that stuff," he said.

"PloughShare?" said the television woman. "A charity?"

"Based in Ethiopia," I said.

"Oh." She was dark and pretty. Her eyes had been shining at me as if I was the lens of a camera. They stopped shining. "We did a whole lot of stuff on Ethiopia . . . was it ten years back?"

"Who knows?" said her cameraman. "I was in college, I guess."

They asked a couple more questions. Then they filed out, still with the shallow grins pegged to their faces. I lay there in the room with the TV, the telephone and the bowl of fruit. I thought: Devis, you are out of your depth. Your sister has been shot with her husband who is a household name in America. You go abroad seeking publicity for your cause. Your boat is sunk under you, and your crew is machine-gunned. And you get twenty seconds on TV and three inches on page seven of a small-town newspaper. If you want to make it up to the memory of these people, you are going to have to do better than that.

The door opened and a head came around. It was a big head, or maybe it was only the hair that made it look like that. There was a lot of hair, blackish and grizzled. There was also a lot of beard. What skin was visible was the color of a distressed elm sideboard. The eyes were black, suspicious and sharp. The head said, "You George?"

I said, "That's right."

A body followed the head. It was wide and flat, dressed in a dark blue welder's boiler suit. Around the right wrist was a watch strap consisting of the most elaborate Turk's head I had ever seen. On the feet were a pair of deck shoes brought by age and wear to resemble giant samosas. From rents in their fabric were escaping numbers of unclean toes. He said, "I'm John."

I said, blankly, "John." He looked like someone who had stepped into the hospital room halfway through sailing across the Pacific.

"Scotch John," he said. "I knew Rhyd."

I said, "Oh." I had never heard of him. Scotch John sniffed, took a banana from the bowl and began to eat it, having apparently forgotten I was in the room.

I said, "So what can I do for you?"

He finished the banana, pulled a length of cord out of his pocket, and began knotting. His fingers were as thick as crowbars. An elaborate knot began to grow. "About the boat," he said, eventually.

"What about the boat?"

"Rhyd's dead," he said. "He always told me: Anything happens, George Devis gets the boat. He's the only one interested."

"*Halcyon*," I said.

"That's right," said Scotch John. "Nice boat."

A silence fell. After Camilla and the boys, *Halcyon* had been my chief link with Rhyd. It was *Halcyon* we had been talking about on that last night. And we had sailed together, up the English Channel and into the North Sea: Rhyd and Camilla and I running *Auk* and cooking, watch and watch, while Mary Morpurgo complained about the rain and read books and, when in the mood, ambushed me in the hot, slippery forepeak.

I had only seen the pictures of *Halcyon*, but the pictures were pretty. She was forty-one feet long, a ketch, built of larch on Canadian rock elm frames. She had fast, old-fashioned lines, and she was sound as a bell—or so Rhyd had said. Under the terms of the will, she was mine.

One boat goes down. Another boat comes up. The rewards of cowardice.

Scotch John was watching his fingers as he worked at his rope. It seemed to be a square sinnet lanyard with an intricate knob knot on the end. There was a massive solidity about him that went strangely with the delicate knot. I got the feeling that, left undisturbed, he would sit there fiddling away until somebody asked him to go somewhere else.

I was wrong.

He gave me a sharp, surprisingly shrewd look over his beard. He said, "You sellin' the boat?"

I said, "I don't know."

"Sure," he said. He allowed his eyes to rest on me. "I guess you're sick, at that. Get well. Boat's at Quogue, Maine. Hundred miles up the coast from here." He pulled a pen out of his dungarees pocket and wrote an address in neat italic script on the back of an old weatherfax printout. "Keys, mail and groceries at Rooney's Lunch and Lobster. I live down there. I got a kind of tugboat-houseboat in the harbor. I been looking after *Halcyon*. You ever want a crew, I'll crew."

The door opened and the policeman came in. John got up. He looked at me, then at the policeman. He walked through the policeman as if he was not there. "Hey," said the policeman. "Watch—"

But he was gone.

"Friend of yours?" The cop's upper lip was making his moustache writhe.

I said, "I don't know."

The cop stuck his thumbs into his belt and blew a doom-laden sigh through the moustache. "Those pictures your friend took," he said.

"Yes?"

"Fog," said the policeman. "Hunnert percent gray wool. Mr. Devis, you are free to go."

I would have liked to go. I passed out instead.

7

*T*HEY HAD BROUGHT ME A LITTLE BAG OF SHAVING SOAP, RAZOR, toothbrush and aftershave. Next morning, I hauled myself out of bed and used it all except the aftershave. The mirror showed the usual pugilist with a proper transatlantic tan, but with a yellowish look, as if the skin underneath was trying to be white. When glazed with lust, Mary Morpurgo used to say that it was the face of a Greek warrior: Hector or Achilles. But Mary Morpurgo was much given to fantasies in the classical vein. The best you could say for it this morning was that it did not look actively criminal. I hoped that a close observer might have detected gleams of good nature in the bloodshot eyes. On the whole, it looked like the face of a shipwreck victim with rubber knees and a mission.

I pulled on the jeans and T-shirt I had been wearing when the bad things had started to happen, newly laundered. I pulled the credit cards and passports out of the grab bag, checked them over, cut Bill's cards in half. The nurse came in.

She smiled with her beautiful teeth. She said, "I brought you the papers. You were on TV."

"How did it go?"

She said, "You looked like you needed sleep. The way you look now. It wasn't a real big item." She left.

The story was on page seven of the *Intelligencer*. It said that an English yacht had been sunk at sea, that Bill had been killed, and I had survived. The reporters managed to give the impression that it was an uninteresting episode, connected with uninteresting personalities. There was no mention of Plough-Share. I thought: Bill would have known how to handle this. Another triumph for British reserve.

I stayed in the room and ate lunch. I would have liked a beer or two, but they did not have any beer. Then I used the telephone.

First, I rang Jerry Stein at the PloughShare office in Bristol and told him what had happened, in detail. He said, "I can't believe it. What are you going to do?"

I had been thinking about this.

The object had been for Bill and me to do a double act on the lecture circuit. Now Bill was dead, I had the feeling that I was under an obligation to continue as a single act, double power. I said, "Carry on."

Jerry said, "George, are you sure you can hack this?"

I said, "I've done lectures. Poetry readings."

"Don't read them poetry," he said.

He and Bill had worked out a schedule of lectures: not your full-blown coast-to-coast extravaganza-type lecture tour, but about a dozen lunches and dinners in the houses of Bill's better-heeled contacts, at which we had been supposed to tell fat cats and their thin wives about the work of PloughShare. "Trust me," I said, and gave him the hospital's fax number.

He said, "Sure." He still sounded nervous. Like Rhyd and Camilla, he was of the opinion that poets who bred ducks in the wilds of Devon were wasting their lives. Rhyd would have nodded and grinned and expected nothing much. But I had stood in the hot sun in the bitter smell of ashes. I had seen the despair in the face of Esias the silversmith. *Help us*, he had said. *In the name of your sister, and of God.*

And of Rhydian Walters; and Bill Marsden, who had hammered on the door in Devon and got me into this, and arranged the lectures. I could give lectures. I could raise money.

I remembered Camilla on the day I had left school. The headmaster had lectured the leaving contingent on the need for a temperate life, and told us that our best years were already gone. We wandered blinking into the bright day outside the gloomy assembly hall, contemplating a future that would be even less free than school.

It was eleven o'clock. Parents were expected to collect their children at noon. We stood around, flat and dejected.

And there was a sound.

It was the sound of brass instruments playing, far away. The masters scowled. The music grew louder. It was "Colonel Bogey." And it was not a record player.

Around the bend in the drive came two vehicles. The first was a lorry. On the back of the lorry was seated the Pulteney Silver Band, blowing its lungs out.

The second was a Rolls-Royce, mostly covered in flowers. At the Rolls-Royce's helm was Camilla in a picture hat.

The leaving contingent watched with its mouth open as Camilla drew up in front of Big School and deployed the band on the green turf on which nobody was allowed to walk except the headmaster. Camilla said, "Champagne in the boot."

By the time the other parents arrived, the band was playing the "Blue Danube" and Camilla was dancing with the headmaster.

In the Rolls on the way home, I thanked her for this display of extreme courage.

She grinned at me, the old Camilla grin that lit up the car: English rose with thorns. "Least I could do," she said.

Like the lecture tour.

I called England again. I spoke to the headmaster of Joe and Harry's school. He knew the terms of the will. I arranged a flight to Boston for the boys, then I collected the urn and went off to do my duty.

The label said MARIA WALTERS. There was an address on Laurel Drive in Concord, Massachusetts, and a telephone number. It was right and fitting that I should complete Bill's mission.

I dialed the number on the label, which rang, and rang, and rang. It was mid-afternoon, when all self-respecting people would be at work. If Rhyd's sister was anything like Rhyd, she would be a self-respecting person.

The nurse came back. I filled in a lot of forms for her. I shoved the urn in the stained blue holdall and walked with the minimum possible amount of zigzagging to the elevators.

Outside it was a warm May day. The sky was what I had come to think of as Portland blue, and so was the sea, with little white wisps of sail leaning over the water.

I bought a pair of canvas trousers, blue, a couple of T-shirts, blue, and a pair of Docksiders, blue, and shoved the spares alongside Rhyd's ashes in the grab bag. Then I staggered out to the Hertz depot, rented a car, sweated my way on to the Interstate and headed south toward Boston and Concord.

The driving was nice and slow. The car was big. I worked out how to use the cruise control, and kept my foot on the accelerator.

I found I was thinking about Rhyd's family. They sounded a dour, farmerish bunch. It was no surprise that Rhyd barely mentioned them; the only thing that was surprising was that he had wanted the boys to meet them, and that Camilla had agreed.

But then they had taken them to Ethiopia, too. It had always been one of Camilla's basic notions that all experience was good experience.

After an hour, I stopped at a restaurant and ordered a cheeseburger. The woman in the white overall asked me if I was Australian. The burger tasted of gray gristle. Green signs crowded in on the road. I turned west on 95, squinting at the Rand McNally road atlas in the passenger seat.

Concord was a few miles west of Boston along Highway 2. I passed signs to Walden Pond. The road was quiet in the gray dusk, winding among maple woods that shut out the low evening light with their foliage. There was fog in the air. The houses became small and close together. I counted the numbers on the mailboxes. Number sixty-four was small and square, built of white clapboard and set back from the road. It had a no-messing tarmac garden and a satellite dish. Smoke leaked from an incongruously fat fieldstone chimney. I hoisted the bag on to my shoulder, walked rubber-legged to the front door and pushed the entryphone button.

A woman's voice said, "Who's there?"

"George Devis."

"Who?"

"Rhyd's brother-in-law. Bill Marsden gave me your address."

"Oh." There was a pause. A light went on over the door. There was a spyhole. The entryphone said, "Come right in."

The door opened. I went in.

It was a white, boxy hall, with golden floorboards I recognized as maple. Standing on the boards was a slim woman with short, curly hair that just escaped being red, and slanted eyes that were just the gray side of green, and white skin freckled like a sandpiper's egg. I stood dead still, staring at her. She was a couple of inches shorter than me, dressed in a baggy blue T-shirt tucked into a pair of baggy khaki canvas trousers. On her right wrist she was wearing a Mickey Mouse watch.

She had been staring at me, too. She said, "Are you okay? You look kind of . . . well, blasted." She had a hoarse, breathy voice that sounded less in control than she looked.

"Blasted," I said. "That's it."

"You want a drink?" she said.

"Beer," I said. I wanted an excuse for sticking around.

She went into the back of the house. I heard the noise of a fridge door open and close. There was a photograph of Bill on the mantelpiece, next to one of Rhyd wearing a Stetson, playing a big Gretsch Tennesseean on stage. She came back with two Bud Lites and led the way into a room with three sofas in front of a fire of logs. Her waist was narrow. She said, "My roommate's in Europe." Her voice was faintly nervous, as if she was trying to fill the silence.

I sat on the sofa and took a sip of beer, and gripped the grab bag. A guitar leaned against a chair, a Japanese Martin copy. A Macintosh glowed on a table by the window. There was a pile of spiral-bound notebooks beside the computer, and a pocket tape recorder.

She said, "So you were there when it . . . happened. Both times."

I said, "Happened?" My throat felt as if someone had slammed a safe door down there, and spun the tumblers, and I did not know the combination.

"First Rhyd and your sister. Then Bill." She had a smile that showed nice teeth; not dramatic like the nurse's, but nice all the same. Her face had a taut look: prominent cheekbones, a big clean jaw. Her eyes were unnervingly slanted, the left more steeply than the right. It was a clever face, made more so by the fact that she seemed to be watching you from two directions at once. It was also a face that looked as if it was meant to be funny. But it was not happy. Above the smile, the lower lids were damming up tears.

She said, "It's great you came." She lit a cigarette. "I don't really smoke," she said.

I shrugged.

"Tell me," she said.

I watched her closely. I said, "There's not a lot to tell. It was quick."

She said, "You don't want to talk about it."

"That's right."

"How about the kids?"

"They're coming over. I'm meeting them at the airport tomorrow."

"Oh?"

"To stay with . . . your sister."

She nodded and pitched the half-smoked butt into the fire. "I'll have to get around her, go visit." She sighed. "It's unbelievable," she said. "Across the *Atlantic,* for Christ's sake. And some drug smuggler sinks him . . . you . . . fifty miles off the coast of the United States. Shitty little story, page eight of the *Globe*. And that's all."

She sounded sad, and disappointed. I could not tell whether it was because of Bill's death or the size of the newspaper story.

"That's all," I said.

"And you've been in the hospital, in shock?"

"That's right."

"I guess that wouldn't help your memory."

I sipped beer. I said, "Things are a little hazy."

"And the ashes." She said the word as if she did not want to pronounce it.

The urn was smooth and hard in the bag under my arm. I frowned. I said, "Ashes?"

"Bill was bringing me an urn. Rhyd's ashes."

I said, "I don't know anything about any ashes. I'm afraid they must be on the bottom of the sea."

She said, "Oh, good *grief*." She sounded more cross than upset; as if the ashes had an actual as well as a sentimental value.

"But he sent his love."

"He did?"

"Just before he . . . died." It was a lie. What he had said was *bag label*.

Her face softened. A tear rolled out of each gray-green eye, ran down each freckled cheek, and made a dark spot on each khaki knee.

I said, "I'm sorry."

She smiled. She said, "I guess we were both good friends of Bill. It's so hard to believe." She drew a deep breath. "You want to stay for dinner? We could talk. I made some kind of stew."

I got up. My knees were even rubberier than before. I said, "Thank you, but I've got some people to see."

She said, "It was kind of you to call by." She pulled a card from her pocket. "If you want me, here I am. You could need some help with the kids, right? I'd love to meet them."

I nodded and grinned out of a face that felt like wood. She showed me out of the door.

We drove away up Laurel Drive, me and Rhyd's ashes. I was sweating.

From the little Rhyd had told me about his sisters I knew there was Sarah, who was widowed and lived on the family farm at Bethel Bay; and there was Maria. Maria had kicked against the grim, thick-headed religion of their upbringing and run away a couple of years before Rhyd had taken his guitar on the road. He had not seen her since. He had showed me a picture of her once. She must have been about ten when the picture had been taken. She was a tall girl, golden-skinned, with twin bunches of blond hair and cornflower blue eyes that turned down at the corners.

People change over the years. But their skins do not change from golden to freckled, and their eyes do not turn from blue to gray-green and change their tilt.

The woman who had given me a beer and asked for Rhyd's ashes had been kind and considerate. Under other circumstances, she would have been a woman I could have liked getting to know. She had been smart, and she had been attractive.

But she had certainly not been Rhyd Walters's sister.

8

OUTSIDE LAUREL DRIVE I GOT LOST ALMOST IMMEDIATELY. I DROVE out of the trees and the historic sites until Boston reached out to grab me. A red neon motel glowed in the foggy dark. I ate something they called a Caesar salad in a restaurant with gingham tablecloths, had more beers, and checked into the motel.

It was a big, seedy cabin, a nonsmoker that stank of old cigarettes. For a moment I almost wished I was back in hospital. But only for a moment. I lay on the bed and did battle with the revisitations of the Caesar salad, and watched the red light of the sign on the grubby curtains.

There was a telephone directory by the bed. There was no Maria Walters listed on Laurel Drive. Assume the supposed Maria Walters was a country and western fan, wishing to get hold of her hero's remains. She had known Bill, for sure. She had been much more interested in him than in Rhyd. It looked very much as if Bill had cooked up the Maria story. The real Maria was still off the map. But why bother? And why address the urn to an impostor?

There was as much fog inside my head as outside the hotel room. I fell asleep.

Next morning, I woke with a headache made up of bad food and worse ventilation. I showered and went looking for Logan Airport.

The traffic thickened as I met the queue for what turned out to be the Sumner Tunnel toll. I was able to stop concentrating on navigation and take time to think.

What we had was a little urn, soldered tight, containing bone splinters, wood ash and a couple of pinches of Ethiopian soil. All of which were thought to be important, at any rate by Bill, who had gone to the trouble of collecting them and directing them to a false address.

When I had got the boys organized, I would have to come back to Concord and ask some direct questions.

They came out of the arrivals gate side by side, shepherded by a blond stewardess. Joe was taller than the stewardess. He was pale, deeply conscious of his dignity as a teenager, but allowing his eyes to skid around him at the fascinations of a big airport. Harry was reading Terry Pratchett. When away from natural history items, Harry was usually to be found in a book. Terry Pratchett was his current enthusiasm.

When they saw me, their faces came alight in gratifying style. "You got here!" said Joe.

"Bloody miracle, if you ask me," said Harry.

They had picked up hints of their parents' view of my general usefulness. I was simultaneously touched and mortified. I said, "We sank the boat."

Joe said, "We heard. It was in the *Daily Mail.*" His face was serious. "Jolly bad luck."

Harry looked as if he wanted to make a joke, but had thought better of it. He was chewing bubble gum, against regulations. I got it spat out, bought them a hot dog and sweets for the trip, frog-marched them out to the car, loaded up the luggage, and pointed the nose toward Maine.

There was the usual roar of conversation. Joe had been building a marsh buggy in the school welding shop. Harry had hatched twenty-six bantams in the school incubator. They wanted to know about the air-sea-rescue helicopters. But underneath it all was a nervousness. None of us had met Sarah Walters. We were all on the lip of the unknown, at a moment when things needed to be as normal and reassuring as possible.

We were, however, in America.

Harry gaped at a plywood square-rigged ship in a used car lot beside Highway 1. He said, "Weird."

Joe said, "Snob." He said it for the sake of saying it, the same way Harry had said it was a miracle I had made it to the airport. Joe was worried, and so was Harry. That made three of us.

There was a silence that lasted fifty miles. Finally, Joe said, "What's this old bat like?"

It was not necessary to be psychic to realize he was talking about Sarah. I said, "She lives on a farm."

"Yes," said Joe. There was a pause. "Well, I suppose there'll be tractors." Tractors were one of Joe's enthusiasms.

"And ducks," said Harry.

There was another silence. Some miles of freeway unrolled under the car's yellow bonnet.

Harry said, "Why couldn't we stay with you?" in a voice that was smaller than usual. "It's not fair." He was sticking his jaw out in order not to cry. He had had a lot to cry about, these last four months.

"Your dad wanted to give you a chance to see where he was born. Try it out, see if you like it."

"We've hardly even heard of her. We don't know her."

I said, "She's your aunt."

"But we don't *know* her."

"She'll be terrific."

"And there's the son," said Harry. "Chuck. Dad said he was weird, once."

"He's your cousin," I said. "This place is bang on the sea. You'll be fine." I realized I was more hopeful than confident. Rhyd had severed all connections with the Brethren, but the ties must have been powerful for his sister to feature so prominently in his will. He had said as much, one of the only times he had mentioned it. "Worst thing," he had said, "isn't that they want you back. It's that they can make you want them want you back."

So here I was, delivering the boys to a stranger. Last night I had failed to deliver their father's ashes to a stranger. It was the kind of thing that would have amused Camilla. You hang on to the things that don't matter, and give away the things that do.

"Anyway," I said. "Sarah'll be terrific, or your dad wouldn't have sent you here." I was talking to myself.

Sixty miles north of Boston, the highway bypasses Portland and heads east, shrunken now, following a coast that becomes increasingly ragged, indented with bays and sounds and drowned river valleys as it approaches the Canadian border.

Soon after we crossed the Maine state line, the fog came in again. Both the boys slept. We drove through a country of black pines and ghostly maples. The woods had wisps of gray mist caught in the trees. East of Ellsworth the houses became smaller. A lot of the bigger ones had a shuttered look, as if they were holiday cottages not yet open for the season. The smaller ones had piles of lobster pots, clapboard-patched with sheets of shuttering ply. The only things that shone were the pickup trucks.

We stopped for a final Coke in Red Hill. The woman in the diner had a Belfast Marine cap, size twenty-two ski pants and two tiers of chins. There was a television turned up earsplittingly loud, fishing baits and chainsaw oil behind the bar. "Fog," said the fat woman. "Famous for it, state of Maine. Don't usually get it this early in the year. But we got it, all right."

Joe, in an access of bravery, said, "We're coming to live here."

The woman's chins shifted themselves into a huge smile. "Zat so?" she said. "Where's that?"

"Bethel Bay," said Joe. "Mrs. Ebden."

Her grin stiffened. "Sarah Ebden," she said. "You the Walters boys?"

"That's right," said Harry.

"Real sorry to hear about your dad," said the woman.

Harry's shoulders squared. He had been extremely proud of his father's fame. "Are we near?"

"Five miles," said the fat woman. "Nearest store there is."

"Well," said Harry, with the air of a prince bestowing a "By Appointment" certificate, "we'll be buying our sweets . . . candy here from now on."

The fat woman wagged her head. "Sure," she said. "The name's Daisy Rider."

They shook hands with her, staring her straight in the eye. She reached up to a shelf, puffing. "Here's a Hershey bar," she said. "I guess you never had one before."

"Never," they said.

"Be seein' you," she said.

We left. I thought about the way her grin had left her.

A mile out of town, we turned off the blacktop on to a road of oiled dirt that snaked between two stony hills and sank into a white bed of fog from which black pines jutted like teeth.

"Like Narnia," said Harry.

"Wicked witch and all," said Joe.

We all laughed. They meant it. I did not.

The track became a succession of holes, linked by banks of boulders that set up an unmusical twanging in the hire car's suspension. There was a pond alongside. Crows rattled out of the trees. After a couple of fields of rushy grass, a clump of maples swam out of the fog. There were hard edges in the trees. Buildings.

"Blimey," said Joe. "It's all wood."

We jounced between a pair of gateposts and into a rough square of buildings, perhaps sixty yards on each side. On the left was a clapboard house. At the far end was a long barn with a shingled roof, the walls painted the color of dried blood. On the right was a shorter barn, two bays knocked out to make a tractor shed, a couple of doves crouched despondingly on the ridge of the hipped roof. In the middle of the yard was a giant maple tree, its stubby trunk supporting an inverted bowl of branches that must have been a hundred feet from side to side.

On the first step of the three heading up the clapboard porch of the house, a woman was standing. She gave no sense that she had come out of the house, or had been going back in. She might have been standing there all afternoon, as much a fixture as the screens or the tree. She had hair that might once have been blond, but was now pale yellow, heavily streaked with gray. Her face was square, the flesh bitten away under high cheekbones. Her eyes matched the gray streaks in her hair. They looked as if they were a fraction of an inch too far open. They were staring at us with alarming intensity from above a thin mouth that did not smile.

I said, "Sarah Ebden?"

"That's right." This time, there was no doubt that this was Rhyd's sister. They had the same bones. In Rhyd, the fleshy covering had made the face strong and welcoming. In his sister, the bones looked harder and more prominent, so the strength turned to obstinacy, and the welcome was diminished.

She said, "You're welcome here." She smiled. It was a kind smile, but she looked as if she did not practice it much.

The boys introduced themselves, ramrod-straight, one megawatt eye contact, as taught by Rhyd. She smiled again, as if it reminded her of something. She said, "Come on in. You'll be tired after your trip."

Harry said, "Where's the sea?"

Joe said, "Have you got a tractor?"

She turned to lead us up the steps and into the house. She might not have heard. Harry made a face at Joe, who shrugged his shoulders and played a couple of bars on an imaginary saxophone. I said, "You can explore later."

The inside of the house was cool; cold, even. There was a big kitchen, with a huge fridge and Formica worktops, and a crewel sampler that said THE LORD GIVETH AND THE LORD TAKETH AWAY. The boys were not looking at the sampler. They were looking at the table, which was covered in food.

A second silence followed the first silence. This one was full of the sound of jaws at work on sausages and bacon, pancakes and maple syrup, and various forms of bun and biscuit. Gaunt her face might be, and grim her taste in mottoes, but the cooking got their attention.

Sarah dealt the stuff on to their plates and kept me supplied with mud-colored tea. Otherwise, she did not speak. Finally, even Harry leaned back in his chair and refused a pancake. Joe said, "Could we have a look?"

"A look?"

"Explore," said Harry. "Snoop. You know."

"Sure," said Sarah. "Only don't go in the end barn."

"Why not?" said Joe, who always needed to know why everything.

"Chuck's sleeping," said Sarah. "Chuck lives down in the barn, and he needs his rest."

"How old's Chuck?" said Joe.

"Seventeen," said Sarah. "He runs the farm."

"Sure," said Joe. He was getting the language already. "Thank you for a most delicious tea."

"Sure," said Sarah, without smiling. "Run along now."

The boys wandered out, studiedly casual. I watched them through the net curtains. Harry spat, the way American farmers spat in his imagination, and began absentmindedly patting an old black-and-white dog that had slunk out of the tractor barn. Joe slid into a shed, no doubt in search of machinery. I said to Sarah, "I hope they're not going to be too much trouble."

She rested her surprised gray eyes on me. "The laborer is worthy of his hire," she said. "There is no trouble in duty."

There was a silence. We gazed out of the window at the huge tree, the blood-colored barn, the black pines in the gray fog. I said, "So this is the family farm?"

"Three hundred and eleven years," she said. "Walterses without a break."

I took a deep breath. "Rhyd spoke of it a lot," I said.

The eyes were chilly and unwavering. "I'm surprised he could remember it," she said. "He forgot so much."

"Forgot?"

"The faith of his forefathers," she said. She was sitting with her hands folded, knees together, legs uncrossed, eyes downcast. All she needed was a Welsh bonnet and a white collar and she could have stepped straight off the *Ark* with the first Brethren. "He turned his back on redemption." She sounded more sad than angry.

I said, "But he loved the farm."

She shrugged. "Lay not up for yourselves treasures upon earth, where moth and rust doth corrupt, and where thieves break through and steal."

I said, "I have his ashes. I think he would have liked them scattered here."

Her face became blank, as if I had said something outrageous. She got up. "Come out here," she said.

She led me out of the house and through an orchard to a small wooden building that crouched on the edge of a grove of ancient maples. The maples were battered and twisted. Through their trunks, an inlet of gray sea muttered on a beach of stones. Around the building was mown grass, green and matted and ancient-looking. In the lawn were many hummocks, six feet long, a foot wide. "Here," she said. "Our Brethren."

The sun was a weak silver eyeball hanging in the mist. The hummocks made faint shadows on the wet sward. "All of them?" I said.

"All of them. John Walters, the firstcomer, on down." She paused. Somewhere in the fog a gull shrieked. "We believe in the corporeal resurrection," she said. "That at the sound of the trumpet, all shall rise again in the body."

So ashes were not much good.

I pointed at the wooden building. I said, "And that's your chapel?"

"That is the House of God."

I have never been able to pass a church without sticking my nose in. I moved across the fog-pearled grass toward the door.

"Stop!" For the first time since I had met her, her voice was full of emotion. "Only the Brethren may penetrate the Tabernacle."

"Oh," I said. "Fine." And we stood there, her getting her feet wet among her ancestors, me feeling an idiot.

Water crunched on the shore of the bay beyond the trees. A duck quacked. A boy started shouting: Harry, laughing like a monkey. "Silly old fool!" he yelled.

"No!" That was Joe. He was not laughing. "Don't!" Then there was another sound: a big explosion. Two explosions.

I knew the sound, from times when I had been stalking red deer in the Highlands of Scotland. Somebody was shooting with a powerful hunting rifle.

I began to run like hell back to the yard.

9

*W*HEN I GOT INTO THE YARD, THERE WAS A LOT OF SHOUTING. There were Joe and Harry, and another voice, loud and flat. "Git away!" it was yelling. "Git away!"

They were standing in a knot at the far end of the yard beyond the huge maple tree: Joe and Harry, and another kid, who could have been seventeen. I slowed down to a walk. The seventeen-year-old was wearing yellow boots and a checked shirt, and a blue basketball cap with a pinched bill pulled down so far on his head that his ears stuck out. He had a long chin and a short nose and flat, suspicious eyes. His mouth hung open. His lower lip was thick, shiny with spit. The eyes flicked between me and the boys and Sarah. He was holding a big Mannlicher hunting rifle, muzzle pointing at the ground.

"Chuck," said Sarah. "What are you doing?" Her voice was suddenly soft and cajoling.

"They got to keep away," said Chuck. "Who is they anyways?" The words came out haltingly, as if muffled by a medium-sized apple in his mouth.

"These are your cousins," said Sarah. "Joe and Harry. I told you. And this here is your . . . kind of cousin George."

Harry said, "He shot the poor pigeon." He held out his hands. There was a heap of gray feathers, heavily stained with blood. A deer rifle at close range will more or less vaporize a mourning dove.

Sarah said, "What did you do that for, honey?"

Chuck's eyes resumed their patrol. "Too close," he said.

"Okay." She turned to Joe and Harry. "Chuck likes to be private," she said. "You have to keep away from his barn. It's like, everybody has their special place? Their room? Here, I'll show you your rooms." Her voice was still soft. "And Chuck, you put that rifle right back in the cabinet, and I don't want to hear it again."

Chuck nodded. Music was filtering into the shadows under the tree: Rhyd music. It was the tune I had heard him record in Africa on the last night.

I said, "That's your uncle."

A gleam of something that might have been interest appeared in Chuck's eyes. He jacked the cartridges out of his rifle. "Sure," he said. "Rhyd Walters. He's famous."

The boys were talking to Sarah now. Everything had gone normal again, or as normal as it could be. I remembered the brown-paper parcel Rhyd had given me as I had left, that last day. There had been a dozen parcels. I said to Chuck, "He sent you that tape. I posted it from London."

"Yeah," he said. He was looking almost animated. "I love that music. You wait here."

He turned and trotted off, rifle trailing around the end of the barn. When he came back, he had a big book under his arm. "My stamps," he said.

He made me go through it with him. He pointed out the English stamps, the Ethiopian stamps. "Valuable as heck," he said. "Worth a lotta money." There was an engaging earnestness about him as he looked sideways at me, gauging exactly how impressed I was.

"Certainly are," I said. Poor Chuck, I thought. Ten-year-old mind stuck in a seventeen-year-old body.

He said, "I had to show 'em." He was frowning. "Them kids. My cousins."

I nodded. I said, "They've got the message."

He nodded, man to man. "Gun's back in the cabinet now. Locked."

"Sure."

He stumped back to his barn. I was feeling better; not great, but better. I wished that Rhyd were here to look at the place he had condemned his children to. I wished that Camilla were here, to talk to him straight as only she knew how. But then I always wished that Camilla were here.

"C'mon, you folks," said Sarah. She had lost her stiffness. We went back to the house and she showed the boys their rooms, in a little one-story wing at the back, away from the yard. She had done her basic research. Harry had a stuffed deer's head, and Joe had a John Deere tractor calendar. That helped. There were a couple of old bicycles in a shed. That helped, too. Rhyd's guitar drifted through the branches of the tree, a track I did not recognize, with a banjo part. "Chuck," said Sarah. "I'm sorry. He's real stirred up. He took it real hard, about Rhyd. He does love Rhyd's music so. Rhyd was real good to him."

I tried to look interested. Sarah had her soft side, and she seemed kind enough. But I had lived twenty yards away from Joe and Harry for the first five years of their lives. I went back into the wing. I said to Joe, "Are you going to be all right here for the summer?"

"Sure," said Joe. "It's the seaside, innit?"

"Food's all right," said Harry, sticking out his chin in a way that reminded me horribly of Camilla deciding it was her duty to do something she did not want to do.

"And maybe later on you get to fire guns," said Joe. "What I says is, why not?"

"Which is what I says," said Harry.

And there we all stood, sticking our jaws out and being British. I was thinking: This is definitely not right. But it was what had been arranged by their parents. So I kissed them goodbye, and walked to the front of the house where Sarah was waiting.

"Well," I said, with a cheerfulness I definitely did not feel. "You've got some new family." She smiled. "By the way," I said. "Your sister Maria. I should visit her."

She looked at me with eyes suddenly cold as oysters. She said, "I never had a sister called Maria."

I was disconcerted. I said, "Rhyd talked about her."

She stood for a moment. She said, "What my brother talked about was his own affair." She put her finger on her lip, to show that she was thinking. "I'll show you something," she said. She went out of the room.

She came back carrying a leather-bound Bible the size of a suitcase. It had brass corners and a lock. She unlocked it with a key she carried on a chain, and turned the flyleaf. "Look there," she said.

Written in brown-black ink on foxed vellum was what looked like the Walters' family tree. The bottom line but one bore Sarah's name, and Rhydian's and Maria's. Rhydian and Maria had been crossed out with one firm stroke of a pen. The black ink had turned slightly rusty with age.

Chuck's name was on the bottom line. And there were two entries in newer ink than the crossings-out above: Joseph and Henry. The lines connecting them to the tree led firmly not to Rhyd's name, but to Sarah's.

I met her eyes. They were gray and stubborn.

She said, "My family are children of the Lord. When one strays from the strait way of the Lord, they are no family to me."

I said, "Where does your sister live?"

She said, "I am not aware of anything concerning Maria Walters. Now it would be fitting if you would leave."

I said, "I'll say goodbye."

"Best not upset them." She laid her bony hand upon my arm. "I can see you love those guys," she said. "Do me the credit of realizing I love them too."

I should have taken them away then and there. Camilla

would have done. But Camilla had been their mother. And I was only their fifty percent legal guardian, and Sarah was the other fifty percent.

So I walked out into the yard, and I waved, and I drove up along the track and through the pines toward the blacktop road that snaked away through the rocky woods toward Highway 1.

And I left them.

Relax, I told myself. They are going to spend six months on a farm by the sea. Sarah might be odd, and Chuck not bright, but the food is terrific. There are bicycles, and a sweetshop up the road. There had been people with high-powered rifles in Ethiopia. Camilla had said it to me, the first time I had gone out to visit, when I had asked if she did not think it was dangerous: *Why would anyone want to shoot a couple of kids. Us, yes. But why the kids?*

I smelled once again the bad, bitter smell of ashes, felt the sun like a red-hot anvil on my neck, remembered the terror. I took a deep breath. The boys would be fine. I had a debt to pay to Camilla, and the village.

The track was flattening out now. A car was parked ahead, near the shut up holiday cottage where the track joined the road. It had Massachusetts number plates. I went past, turned left, headed back for civilization.

The lecture schedule Jerry Stein had faxed to me in hospital was in my pocket. It said the first speaking engagement was in Lexington, Massachusetts, tomorrow night. The Rand McNally told me Lexington was embedded in Greater Boston. I had to get ready, now that there was no Bill to show me the special skills involved in twanging the heartstrings of the rich. And while I was there, I would pay a visit to the false Maria Walters.

So I drove south and west, down the coast. At eight o'clock the fog was turning brown with dusk, and I was hungry. Over on the right, a sign was yelling RESTAURANT in red neon. I pulled over, parked the car in a big grit car park, and went inside.

They put me at a seat by the window. I ordered a steak and a Bud Lite. The reflections of the diners swam in double exposure over the headlights on the road. There were half a dozen cars in a big car park. I put my forehead against the cold glass, and looked harder.

My car was in the far corner of the car park. Someone was moving over there. There was a figure alongside the driver's door, hunched, as if it was fiddling with the handle. I got up and ran for the exit.

The night air was raw with fog. Grit crunched under my shoes as I ran. The figure was still by the driver's window. The shoulders were moving as if the hands were performing a mechanical operation.

I had never been able to see Mary Morpurgo's point when she called me half-commando, half-hermit. But Camilla had once had an inexplicable boyfriend called Dave, a stocky man of pronounced right-wing views who had done time in the SAS. She said his politics did not matter because they were silly and besides, he was sweet. Dave had taught me to fight, because fighting was all he knew how to do on long afternoons when there was no beer to drink. Go in first, he had said. Go in to kill.

The figure was upright now, hand in the coat pocket. I jumped, grabbed for the neck. We went down in the gravel. I got my forearm around the throat.

There was something wrong.

The neck was too slender. The hair against my face smelled too good. I relaxed my hold.

"Shit," said the voice.

A woman's voice. The voice of the supposed Maria Walters.

I felt the blood rush to my face. I am not the kind of person who makes a specialty of flattening women with flying tackles. I said, "Are you all right?"

She drew back her arm, as if to clout me. She seemed to change her mind. She said, "Good *grief.*"

I looked down at the driver's window of the car. I saw a wire coat hanger, bent straight, rammed between the glass and the rubber seal. Bloody hell, Devis, I thought. She was trying to break into your car, and you ask her if she's all right, and she acts as if you are in the wrong.

Camilla would have laughed herself sick, and been confirmed in her prejudices.

The woman scrambled to her feet and slapped at the grit on her jeans. I said, "What are you doing?"

She said, "Breaking into your car. You know, I think I need a drink?" She turned away. Her shoulders were tight and hunched.

I said, "I'm calling the police."

She said, "I'll be having the drink." She walked away. She turned and looked back. "Maybe we should talk about it." She had a model's walk, one foot in front of the other. She radiated a sort of confidence.

I looked at the car. She had not got in. It would be a hard thing to prove, if she denied it, which she would. She wanted me to talk. I pushed the dirt off my knees and went after her.

She was sitting at my table, sucking her hand. "You cut my knuckle," she said.

The waitress came. The woman ordered a bourbon and club soda. The waitress brought the drink and my steak. I started to eat it.

I said, "What's your name?"

"Ricky Lee Klaasen."

I said, "Why did you call yourself Maria Walters?"

She said, "I used to room with her."

"You what?" It was a shock. I was beginning to believe she really had never existed.

"Room. Share a house. My house in Concord. She was a singer. Sometimes I work as a singer. We sang together."

"So where is she?"

She twiddled the straw in her drink. She wore a ring that might have been glass, or a large emerald. Her fingers were flat ended, with guitar player's callouses. "She left," she said. "She drank, Okay? Not that I mind if people drink. I drink myself. Also, I break into cars. I do all kinds of weird stuff. But Maria had . . . this religious background. You know?"

I knew.

"So she felt bad about drinking. Specially when she couldn't find the strings any more. Kept pulling these clinkers, you know? I told her I didn't mind." She sighed. "But she took herself off. We were playing the Golden Horseshoe in Toronto, Canada. Had a room on Queen Street someplace. I had a date with a guy, nice guy, film maker—they all make films in Toronto. And when I got back to the room, Maria was gone. She left a note. That's all, folks. And . . ." She twiddled the straw. "Well. She was the one who could sing. She played nice flatpicking guitar, nice banjo. I kind of moaned along, played basic guitar, wrote some lyrics. So I pulled the ol' horns in." She sighed. "It was fine," she said. "I returned to the mainstream of my career path." She made a wry face. "Then some lady called, a couple months later. I'd been looking for Maria all over. The lady said she fell under a truck in Canada. I was real sad." Her eyes rested on me. They were kind eyes, and humorous. "I never even found out where they had the funeral." She sighed. "Everyone dies. So I came back, started to scratch me a living in New England."

I did not want to get involved in her hopes and fears. I said, "Tell me about the ashes."

"Bill told me that he'd label the urn with the Maria name, because it might look weird, bringing an urn of ashes across to someone who wasn't family, you know?"

I sawed up some more steak. Weird summed it up neatly. I said, "Why do you want an urn of ashes of someone you don't know?"

"I was on a story with Bill."

"You're a journalist?"

"Boston *Echo*," she said. She stole one of my French fries. The slanted eyes looked away from mine, as if the idea made her uneasy.

I said, "So what was the story?"

"Something about Africa. Something political. Bill talked to Rhyd Walters a lot. When Maria was here, I introduced her to Bill. She wasn't seeing much of Rhyd any more. Bill was . . . some kind of go-between. He'd lifted a corner of some rug or other. He was bringing something back that would roll it up."

I thought about Bill, the perfect crew and partner, always reliable, never asking for anything, never giving anything away. I said, "So what were you doing?"

She laughed and made a wry face. She said, "Pursuing a career in journalism. Ricky Lee Answering Machine. Ricky Lee Maildrop. I didn't open the letters or listen to the calls. This was a big story. Pulitzer big, he said. I asked questions, sure. He didn't answer them. If I pressed him, he said he'd fire me. I don't think he was joking."

"Fire you?"

"I . . . when I said I worked for the *Echo* I guess I was kind of exaggerating a little," she said. "You can work on small-town papers for so long. Then you go to one salad social too many, and you are running boiling apeshit on Main Street. And you can do TV, but I have these funny eyes and I guess my tits are not big enough." She grinned at me and at herself. "And radio sucks, and so does PR. So I decided I would go after a job on a real paper. I met Bill at some party in a gallery. And I worked as his research assistant, except that as you know he didn't tell anyone anything so there wasn't a hell of a lot of research to do. But I got to know the people on the *Echo.*" She finished her drink. "And I thought I would take a look at Bill's evidence, and see if I could take this story of his any further." She spread her hands. "So shoot me," she said. "I hitched a ride with Bill because I needed a break."

"What were you going to do with the ashes when you got them?"

"Take them to the editor of the *Echo.* Bill said."

"Bill said?"

She looked down. Her face was grim. I could see little

brackets at the corners of her mouth, as if she were walking a sharper knife edge than she had admitted. "He called from England. He said he was coming back with an urn. He said that if . . . he fell overboard, the urn would come to me. He was addressing it to Maria, because people would expect an urn of ashes to go to the sister of the . . . deceased. It would look natural, right?"

I nodded. It had looked natural, until Ricky Lee had opened the door.

"So when I got the urn, I should take it to the editor of the *Echo.*"

I pushed my plate away. I was not hungry anymore. I said, "Was he expecting a problem?"

She said, "Bill would not have told you if he was expecting a train. What he said was, people fall overboard crossing the Atlantic."

The Muzak was tinkling a hellish travesty of "Yesterday." Above the muted horns I could hear the plunge of Bill's head in the sea. I buried the sound, quickly. I said, "And would you have handed it over?"

She propped her chin on her hands and looked at me with her slanted greenish eyes. She said, "I hadn't decided. I have my career to think about. I'm a reporter, not just a research assistant." She smiled. It was a quick, intimate smile. "Now, about you. I like the poetry. And I guess that writing books about birds is one of those things someone has to do."

I sipped beer. She was trying to change the subject. I said, "Very knowledgeable."

She said, "I got it from *People of Today.* It's not hard. Except it didn't say you were into military-style self-defense."

There is no section in *People of Today* that deals with things taught you by people your sister fancies. I said, "You go around trying to break into cars, you are taking a risk."

She had the decency to blush.

"So maybe I should call your editor and tell him about it."

She said, "If you feel you have to."

I sipped more beer. I could have called the police, but I was curious about her. I said, "So you're swiping human remains for career reasons."

She said, "That sounds not too good."

"That's the way it's meant to sound."

She looked at me with her slanting eyes. "Well, I guess it's true."

"So what's in the urn?"

"Bones, I guess. Listen, this is all crazy. Keep your goddamn urn. Let's talk about you again. Do you know you have a problem?"

She had a talent for catching me off balance. I said, "What?"

"Bill said you were going to do a lecture tour, you and him."

"That's right."

"Do you have a schedule?"

I pulled the paper out of my pocket. She twitched it out of my hand. She sat stroking her chin with her finger as she read, then slapped the schedule down on the table. She said, "If Bill had been here, he could have beaten the drum for you. He was good at that. But there's other stuff now. The whole damn world's gone crazy. Nobody even remembers where Ethiopia is. Hell, most people thought the Gulf War was the Gulf of Mexico."

I said, "It'll be fine." I said it for my own benefit. I was not confident. I was thinking about the bored reporters in the hospital in Portland, the one paragraph on page eight of the Boston *Globe*. From a diner in Maine, America looked much too big to be impressed by British ornithologist-poets appealing on behalf of small villages in unfashionable countries of which it knew little.

She said, "Who's your press agent?"

I said, "I don't need one."

She pursed her lips. "Mrs. Portarlington Elliott," she said. "Queen of Concord. Fifty rich old women. They all want their names in the paper."

I said, "If it's all right with you, I should be moving along."

She shrugged. "Sure," she said. Her eyes rested on me, cool and faintly amused. "Thanks for the drink."

I said, "You're welcome."

"Very fluent," she said.

As I started the car, I saw her in the restaurant, chin on hand at the table by the window, lit like a fish in a glass tank. She waved at my lights, and returned to her thoughts.

I opened the Rand McNally and headed south. Quogue was the other side of Ellsworth, halfway between Bethel and Portland, twenty-five miles off the road to Boston. It was a good time to look at my new boat. But I was not thinking about boats.

Rhyd and Camilla had known they were under threat, and they had not told me. Bill had been working on an African story, pursuant to which he had been to visit Rhyd, too late.

I heard Camilla again, in the cool bedroom, with the sun blazing through the Alleluia Tree outside.

You can't not get involved.

The steak sat like gravel ballast in my stomach as I plowed through the night. Two options. One: give the lectures, make what I could for PloughShare, go home. Two: give the lectures, find out about Bill's story, and why he had been to visit Rhyd.

The shame was making me sweat.

Get involved.

I was off the freeway now, heading through a light haze of fog. Black trees pressed in on the road. I tried to think of things I could tell the luncheon guests of Mrs. Portarlington Elliott, but big, evil thoughts kept shouldering the headings of my speech aside.

I was thinking of the urn and reasons why Bill and Miss Klaasen might have been so interested in it.

Two journalists after a handful of calcined bone.

If that was what was in the urn.

There began to be wooden houses by the road. I passed a gas station and a mill, a wired-off compound with piles of sawdust and a stack of tree trunks. Then there was a street with clapboard houses, a white church with a wooden spire and lights surrounded by hazy yellow aureoles. There were a couple of stores, closed. Ahead was a line of pilings. The headlights flung their shadows across black water. On the corner, yellow light crept from behind gingham curtains, and a sign said ROONEY'S LUNCH AND LOBSTER. Through a gap in the curtains I saw tables and a door marked KITCHEN STAFF ONLY. A jukebox was playing Willie Nelson. I stopped the car and went in.

There were no customers. The jukebox was very loud. On the white tongue-and-groove walls was a framed photograph of Rhyd wearing a ten-gallon hat with a lobster claw in the band. It was signed *Rave on, Danny, Rhydian Walters.* The man behind the little bar had a face the color of double cream, Ronald Reagan hair, and eyes like currants. I said, "Scotch John told me you have the keys for *Halcyon.*"

The man behind the bar said, "What's your name?" His face was as still as a corpse's.

I told him. He put an elbow on the bar, shoved his face close to mine. "So you're the brother-in-law," he said.

"That's right."

The face cracked open in a tremendous grin, revealing perfect false teeth. "Pleastameecha," he said. "Danny Rooney, at your service. We got beer, we got lobstah, we got the phone, we got Yamaha spares. Plus we got your mail, which you ain't got none."

"And the keys."

"And the keys," he said. "That was real bad, what happened to your sister and Rhyd and all. Listen, have a beer." He gestured at the empty bar. "Plenty room. Season don't start till July."

I had made a decision. I wanted to carry the first part of it through, now, before I lost courage. I said, "I'd love to, some other time. I ought to get a look at that boat."

"Sure," said Danny. His face had stilled again. I got the impression he was lonely and wanted company. He pulled a bunch of keys on a cork-ball key ring off a nail behind the door.

"Keys to boat," he said. "And keys to the car."

"Car?"

He grinned, dazzlingly. "It's up in Donny's net shed," he said. "You might as well use it, I guess. Festus'll give you a ride out. Nice to meet you."

Festus was a spotty youth in what seemed to be the regional uniform of baseball cap, plaid shirt and dirty yellow boots. "Walters' boat," he said, and fell silent. He hitched a dory onto the back end of a big punt with an outboard, fired up the outboard, and roared dead straight into the night. Three minutes later we were alongside a white hull. "Here," he said.

I tossed my bag on deck, took the painter of the dory. Festus roared away. I was standing on a timber deck. Main- and mizzenmasts towered into the fog. The hull rocked faintly in the punt's wake.

There had been a photograph of *Halcyon* above the big beam of polished acacia wood that held up the chimney in the house in Ethiopia. She had two masts, a bowsprit, and a big cockpit for drinking beer in. I could not see much of her in the dark, but I knew what to look for.

I unlocked the hatch, shoved it back, climbed down the companionway and lit the lamp. Rhyd had talked about her so much I could have made the tea with my eyes shut. She had been built in the 1920s by a Bar Harbor grandee who had enjoyed winning races. Unlike modern racing boats, she was built for comfort. The saloon was full of the golden glow of varnished maple. There were neat books, deep settee berths, a squeaky clean gas stove on gimbals. The mainmast came through the cabin top, a pillar of golden pine thick as a tree. On the starboard bulkhead was a big, flat box with sign-written letters: KEEP SHUT—SALT-FREE ZONE. The guitar box. Rhyd had explained it all to me in the Ethiopian night, so dry that you could feel your skin crackle when you moved the muscles of your face. There was a dehumidifier, a moisture meter. It was the only way you could take a Martin to sea without it turning into something like a canoe paddle with strings. There was a sheet of paper on the saloon table. It said, *Here it is ready all tanked up, beer and supplies in icebox. See you, Scotch John.* The handwriting was neat italic.

I was light-headed with exhaustion and nerves about the thing I had to do.

I found a toolbox in a locker in the forepeak and hauled it back into the saloon. From the stained bag I pulled out the urn.

I shook it. It made no sound. Its weight ran into my arms. Devis, I thought, are you going through with this?

I laid it on the bunk. There was a narrow groove where the lid joined the body. It was soldered up. I had no soldering iron.

I began to hit it with a clawhammer, sharp blows, the way you hit the lid of a jar of homemade jam that has rusted shut. My mouth was dry and my heart was thumping. The solder began to crack. Little silver crumbs fell on the blue buttoned canvas. Old Rhyd, I thought. The bloody undertaker couldn't even be bothered to do him up in real bronze. Maybe they don't have real bronze in Ethiopia. My palms were sweating. Get a grip, Devis. It's only ashes. Mostly wood ashes, like you said.

The last of the solder cracked. I turned the urn upright on to its base. It looked sad and battered, a pretentious little tea caddy. Nothing to do with Rhyd or Camilla.

Without giving myself time to think, I shoved the flat end of a big screwdriver under the rim and flicked off the lid.

10

*T*HE URN WAS FULL TO THE BRIM. SOME OF WHAT WAS IN IT spilled over and on to the cushions. I said, "Bloody hell," out loud, with no fear of sacrilege. I felt almost pleased, with the hot flush of pleasure that comes when you wake up from a nightmare and you find that your sister is not dead and your nephews have not been confiscated by religious maniacs in a foggy valley of black pines.

Except she was, and they had been.

But the pleasure remained.

Because what was in the urn did not look anything like what I imagined human ashes to be. What was in the urn was a cream-white powder. No, I thought. Surely not drugs.

I lifted up the urn, sniffed it. It had a vague, faintly wholesome smell. Pulteney is one of those places where rich idiots bring big yachts and have nasty parties. At those parties, I have smelled the acetone whiff of cocaine. This was not cocaine. I have never smelled heroin, but I doubted whether heroin would smell wholesome.

So I took a pinch up between finger and thumb, and tasted it.

It was flour. Plain, not self-rising.

I ran the screwdriver through the stuff to see if there was anything hidden in the depths. There was not. Then I pushed the lid back on, stood it on the saloon table, and looked at it.

Why had Bill and Ricky Lee gone to all this trouble over a pound of plain flour?

I locked the urn in the waterproof guitar locker in the saloon. I slept for five hours, badly, and woke to more fog.

The harbor was a gray disk of water closed in by pine-clad rocks. Houses peered out of the pines at thirty odd scruffy lobster boats on moorings. In the middle of the lobster boats floated something that might once have been a tug. That would be Scotch John's tugboat-houseboat. Smoke wisped from a stovepipe and a flock of crossbreed ducks squabbled on a straw-covered pontoon moored alongside. *Halcyon* was the only yacht. I clambered into the dinghy, pulled away from the side, and leaned on the oars. A loon called, a long, sliding whistle. I sat there on the gray water and breathed a couple of times, getting the ozone to the bottom of the lungs. A lobster-boat engine spat black smoke and rattled into life. I converted the last breath into a sigh, and began to pull for the shore.

There were pickup trucks on the quay with stacks of lobster pots in their backs. I asked a man for directions to Donny's shed. He led me up a narrow track. Inside a pair of blue garage doors was a candy-apple red Mustang.

"So," said my guide. "Your sister married Rhyd, that right?"

I told him that was right.

"Poor guys," said the guide. "That was a terrible thing. You takin' the car?"

"Sure," I said.

"You got a rental," the man said. Everyone in Quogue seemed to know everyone else's business. "Outta Portland?"

I told him that was right.

He said, "I'll drop it off, if you want."

I thanked him, handed him the keys. The Mustang wrapped me in a smell of leather and gasoline. I hit the starter. The engine caught with a hard, throaty bellow.

I backed out of the garage and started on the two hundred

odd miles to the greater Boston area, in which was embedded Lexington, Massachusetts, and the house of Mrs. Portarlington Elliott. On the way I thought about an urn of flour that Bill was bringing surreptitiously across the Atlantic, which was going to wrap up a Pulitzer-scale story. I thought about Bill's editor. It would be useful to talk to Bill's editor.

I stopped in Portland and bought a dark blue suit, button-down shirt and discreet tie. Then I climbed back into the car and concentrated on working up a sort of speech. By the time I arrived in Lexington it was almost noon. A gleam of sun was gilding the shrubs the other side of Mrs. Portarlington Elliott's long red-brick demesne wall. The house had a pediment with carved wooden acanthus leaves, supported by Doric columns. It gleamed like a confection of icing sugar at the end of its butter-yellow sweep of gravel.

I parked the Mustang between a Rolls-Royce and a Cadillac. The deal was lunch and a lecture, followed by contributions for PloughShare. If I did it right, Mrs. Portarlington Elliott and her influential friends would alert their husbands, who would add their contributions to the bounty of their wives.

So I straightened the tie and checked the polish of the shoes, and marched in, feeling well dressed but insignificant.

There were twenty-four ladies around half a dozen little round tables under the Italian molded-plaster ceiling in the oval dining room. About twenty of them were alarmingly thin. They were beautifully dressed, discreetly painted, and fragrant to a startling degree. We drank a little Chardonnay and ate a seafood mousse of staggering refinement. After the sociabilities were over, they let in a few press people and I gave a lecture. I kept it factual and impersonal. The ladies wriggled their shoulders under their silk jackets, and smiled their expensive smiles, and pursed their red old lips in horror at appropriate moments. They seemed mildly gratified to hear that signs of democratic government were stirring in Ethiopia, but soil conversion glazed them over. When you have done some public speaking, you can feel when you have got an audience. This lot were semidetached at best.

I finished sooner than I had meant to, with a moving picture of the burned out bungalow and an appeal for their help in raising the PloughShare project phoenixlike from the ashes. In the back of my mind, the voice was back: *You were there*, it whispered. *You were scared, you ran away.*

They clapped politely. A photographer took photographs. I collected donations amounting to a total of $685. Mrs. Portarlington Elliott shook my calloused hand very, very warmly with her thin jeweled one, and thanked me so much for telling my story, which had moved her very deeply. One of the ladies, younger than the rest, who had drunk five glasses of Chardonnay and showed a lot of tongue, gave me her telephone number. I stepped out, slightly dazed, into the foggy afternoon.

I stood in the yellow gravel by the candy-apple-red Mustang, and tried to convince myself that it had gone well. It was not easy. I sneezed. Nature's way of getting perfume out of the nostrils.

A voice said, *"Gesundheit."* It came from the Mustang. Ricky Lee was sitting in the passenger seat, stifling a yawn. She rubbed her unevenly slanting eyes. "Where have you *been?*"

I got in. Short of familiar faces as I was, I was almost pleased to see her. I said, "What are you doing here?"

"I'm press. I was at the back. You were lousy."

The traces of pleasure vanished. But I had a nasty feeling she was right. I said, "How the hell do you know?"

She said, "You picked up, what, seven hundred dollars? They spend that having their roots colored. And they won't be able to remember your name."

I started the car.

She patted my hand and smiled at me. The slanted eyes were more than slightly diabolic. "Listen, you're in a snit. I understand that. I would be. That was a fine speech. Just fine. But Bill would have known the . . . special circumstances, the buttons to push. And he would have had the backup. You don't get through to these people unless they recognize your name, right? Give me a ride downtown?"

She talked confidently, on home ground. I knew she was right. Bill would have been pulling strings like a champion bellringer. George Devis did not know where to begin.

I stamped on the throttle. The Mustang spewed gravel and whacked us back in the seats. I burnt rubber into the road.

She said, "You think that because you sail this race, you get half killed, this gives you some kind of claim on the attention of the great American public? Bullshit. But you've got a message, and you can talk. I'd like to take you to see somebody who could raise all this to a different level."

I was thinking about Esias and the hot mud streets of the village. I was thinking about seven hundred dollars, the difference it would make. Seven hundred dollars was as much as the village earned in a good year. I looked at her. I thought: You do not know anything. You are in this for your story, not Esias and the village.

"Trust me," she said. "You'll be glad you did."

Trusting her was the problem, but there were only two choices. Trust her, or walk away. I had already tried walking away.

She said, "This is the guy Bill would have plugged into. At least see him."

I passed a taxi on the inside, dived down an exit that said BOSTON. "Who is he?" I said.

She said, "Pierce Rapaport. Editor-in-Chief of Poliakoff Communications Corporation, which owns the Boston *Echo* and a hundred other newspapers, and ten TV stations, including News Actuality. As I have already explained to you, I am trying to continue my career as a reporter, which means bringing in stories, even if they are about Limey creeps. I don't know Pierce real well, but I met him at a party Bill took me to."

I looked at her sideways. "News Actuality?" I said.

"Among others."

News Actuality had been in Baghdad during the bombing, in the crater of Vesuvius during the eruption, and in the coca fields of Peru with the Sendero Luminoso. Even I knew that

News Actuality was the big league. I said, "How are you going to do this?"

She put her hand on my shoulder, as if testing to see if I was solid. She said, "Relax. I know how this organization works. We'll get some people interested in you."

I said, "Another triumph."

She laughed. She said, "College newspaper, Arkansas. Ricky Lee, arts editor, spills coffee on Tom Wolfe's white suit. Macon, Georgia, *Herald Examiner*. Ricky Lee, cub reporter, knocks a front cap off of Kim Basinger with tape recorder mike during limo-back interview on bumpy road. Red Dog, Omaha, *Post*. Ricky Lee arrives for interview with senator, catches him with his dick out and two pompom girls spread across the bed like peanut butter. Senator owns Red Dog, Omaha, *Post*." She paused. "Then Bill took me on and I thought: It's all coming good." She smiled. Her eyes fizzed with real amusement. "So you're not interested in my career. So use me, Devis."

I said, "Bill wanted you to take the ashes to the editor of the *Echo*."

She said, "Yeah." She looked down at her hands. "Howard Sullivan. Howard got a new job."

"So who's the new editor?"

"Lenny Gold. Lenny doesn't know anything about it. I guess Howard doesn't either. Bill used everybody as safe-deposit boxes."

I frowned. I knew enough about journalists to know that Pulitzer-sized stories were of interest to editors.

She sighed. "That was the big problem, working with Bill. He liked to have it all together before he handed over to anyone."

"So you don't know anything about whatever it was he was working on."

She smiled. She said, "How long did you know Bill?"

"Three months."

"Did he have any brothers or sisters?"

"I don't know."

"Where was he from?"

"He didn't say." We were at a set of traffic lights on the edge of the downtown Boston massif. Beyond a jungle of green-painted steel girders, the road ran long and straight under a marine blue sky.

"There you go," she said. "I met him at a party five years ago. I was doing a little, like, networking. Then he called last year, said I could do research for him. The research was all taking phone messages. He was on it for six months, I guess."

"But Sullivan would know."

She pushed out her lips. "Maybe, maybe not," she said. "He was another maildrop, was all. The times I met him, he was cursing Bill out on account of he never told him anything."

The light changed. I drove on. I was thinking about a man you spend all that time with, who does not give you even the vaguest hint that he is shipping urns of flour across the Atlantic in your boat. Never mind why.

I said, "We should find Mr. Sullivan."

She looked back at me, straight-faced. She said, "That is a brilliant idea."

We were heading down a wide road lined with fish markets. There was water on the left, black and dirty, with cardboard boxes floating. Lines of fishing boats lay alongside. Behind us, the towers of downtown Boston bristled. Ahead was a big, luminous sky over an evening sea.

I was wondering about fishing boats. I was wondering about accidental encounters with drug runners, who machine-gunned you and ran you down. Try this, I thought. Two facts. Camilla and Rhyd get killed by an Ethiopian bandit called Ras Hamil. Bill, a confidant of Rhyd's, gets murdered by a scallop dragger a hundred miles south of Cape Sable. Establish a connection.

Not many Ethiopian bandits have access to scallop draggers.

I said to Ricky Lee, "The fishing boat that sank my boat."

"Outside territorial waters," she said. "Could have been anyone. No number, no flags, no nothing."

"You sure?"

She sighed. "I already spent two days on the phone," she

said. "Scallop dragger wanted, repair work to bow sections, at sea ten days ago. They have laughed in my ear all the way from Fort Lauderdale to Virgin's Arm, Newfoundland. No chance at all. Make a left."

I turned along a quay. A couple of hundred yards away, a boat lay alongside. It was an Edwardian steam yacht. It looked as if it belonged in Monte Carlo, not Boston. It was white, with a gleaming black anchor in each hawsehole, a gleaming buff funnel, and a gold-leaf coving line. By the mahogany railed gangway stood a heavily bronzed matelot in white blouse and bell-bottom trousers. At the top of the gangway a mahogany-and-gold-leaf nameboard said *Duchess of Malfi.*

I parked the car. Ricky Lee spoke to the matelot. The matelot spoke into a two-way radio. The radio spoke back.

The yacht towered above us, the size of a young liner. There were radomes and antennae, satellite communications gear nestling among the Dreadnought-vintage details of her upperworks.

"Welcome aboard the *Duchess,"* said the matelot.

I said, "What is this?"

"Global HQ of Poliakoff Communications Corporation," said Ricky Lee.

Serge Poliakoff was the kind of international tycoon whose name had penetrated even into the hills behind Pulteney. He ran a business empire of immense complexity from offices in most of the world's capitals. I had a dim memory of a story in the *Independent,* explaining the means by which he had bought a ready-made newspaper chain on the Eastern seaboard, together with News Actuality. He had declared his intention of beating Ted Turner and CNN on their home ground. The *Independent* had been skeptical about the wisdom of such a move, given the sums of money Mr. Poliakoff had borrowed to make it. I knew nothing about the communications industry, but the *Duchess of Malfi* was certainly an impressive office building.

Ricky Lee squared her shoulders. I followed her up the

gangway. She was wearing a dark blue suit with a shortish skirt and red shoes. Her one-foot-in-front-of-the-other stride had become the hell-with-you strut of a featherweight boxer. We moved along the deck to a varnished mahogany door. The door opened. Another matelot ushered us discreetly along a corridor and through another door.

"Mr. Poliakoff's private offices," said Ricky Lee. She winked at me. Her smile showed traces of nervousness, like a trainee Vestal in the presence of the Sacred Flame.

There was a navy blue carpet deep as a minor sea. On the silk walls were overcleaned Dutch marine paintings that might have been by Van de Velde. The whole place was hot, faintly scented with artificial roses, entirely unboatlike. I found it hard to breathe.

A man was standing in front of a desk. He looked thin and athletic, with a neat, suntanned face and short brown hair. He was wearing a bow tie, gray flannel trousers, a houndstooth-check jacket and loafers that gleamed softly, like the hide of a pedigree stallion. He was looking at Ricky Lee with one eyebrow somewhere close to his hairline.

"Ricky Lee," he said. His voice was light and humorous. "Nice to see you."

Ricky Lee smiled at him, a smile that contained a surprising amount of respect. "Pierce Rapaport," she said. "George Devis."

"Ah, yes," said Rapaport. He turned his needle-sharp brown eyes on me. "George, how are you?" I got the feeling he had known me for years. "The survivor. Welcome aboard the *Duchess.*" He opened a Louis Quinze fridge. I accepted a beer, Czechoslovakian Budweiser. Ricky Lee had a Coke. Pierce had whiskey, Macallan, neat, no ice.

"So," said Pierce. "Ricky Lee tells me it was you sailing with poor Bill." He paused, nose in his glass, looked at me narrowly from the tops of his eyes. "Not an accident, I hear?" he said.

I said, "It was murder, by drug smugglers."

He said, "Stupid way to go."

He made me talk him through the race. His questions were editor's questions, sharp and to the point.

Finally, he said, "We valued Bill Marsden here. He was one of those people who . . . perpetually generate useful ideas. And he won us several major awards in the past. He told me he was on a story before he went to Ethiopia after Christmas."

"That's right," I said.

Pierce said, "Bill liked to keep quiet until he had the overview. I don't know what the story was. If you can help, I'd like to have some people complete the investigation."

I said, "He didn't talk about it."

He sipped his whiskey. He had taken several sips, but the glass was as full as when he had first poured it. He said, "I'm not at all surprised. So you don't know anything at all."

I could have told him it was something to do with a pound of plain flour dressed up as ashes, except that I was not convinced that that had anything to do with it. I said, "Very little."

He said, "I know this much. It concerned events that culminated in the deaths of your sister Camilla and Rhyd Walters."

I had guessed that much. It was nice to have confirmation. It made the shame smaller, more manageable, to know I was still there, on the case. I said, "I know who did that."

"You do?" The eyebrows were up. He might have been asking if I wanted more coffee.

"A man called Ras Hamil," I said. "Or at least, his gunmen. Warlord."

Pierce nodded, as if he knew. He said, "I believe the correct term is prominent figure in emergent democratic grouping."

I was back in the office of the thin colonel in Addis Ababa, the whitewash flakes fluttering in the breeze from the fan, the sweat of shame running inside my shirt.

"And it's a little awkward," Pierce said. "For reasons not connected with the story. You wouldn't consider keeping quiet about this?"

Suddenly the blood roaring in my body, the way it used to

before a race out there on the water in front of Pulteney, when you were on the right side of the course, and it all looked good. These were powerful people, interested in what interested me. They could help me pay back to Camilla some of the things I owed her. *In the name of your sister, and of God.* I said, "Don't be bloody stupid."

He grinned again. This was not the welcome-aboard-the-*Duchess* grin. This was the genuine article. "I'm real happy to hear that. Ricky Lee tells me that you and Bill were planning a lecture tour."

"It's already started."

He nodded. "And you could use some help." He smiled. "I think the least we can do is give you some of that."

I had had limited experience of media big shots since I had given up making wildlife films. What I did have told me that they very seldom performed disinterested acts of charity for foreigners pulled in off the street. I said, "To what do I owe this sudden outbreak of patronage?"

I could feel Ricky Lee freeze. She was not used to people being this blunt with her employers. Rapaport's grin turned even more boyish. He said, "It's not definite yet." He looked around. "There are things that happen in corporations for their own reasons. Just take it that you arrived at a good moment. Can I assume that you are anxious to find out as much as possible about the circumstances in which your sister was killed?"

I said, "Of course."

"And these lectures are intended to raise money for her charity."

"PloughShare."

"PloughShare. This could be real promising." He drummed his fingers on the Morocco desktop. "Thank you for this, Ricky Lee."

Ricky Lee nodded, as if it was all in a day's work, but she could not stop the skin between her freckles turning pink with pleasure.

Rapaport fingered his hatchet jaw. The eyes had become smoky and distant. "The race is over and gone. Bill's murder was two weeks ago. And PloughShare's a British charity. It's not a natural for us. But it can be done, okay. Bill makes a difference."

Ricky Lee said, "The *Echo* doesn't have a campaign right now."

"Africa," he said. "I don't know. There's the firemen's strike in New York City." He picked up a red telephone and murmured something into it. Then he made another couple of calls. He put the phone down. He said, "I think we'd like to use these lectures as a vehicle to . . . commemorate the life and work of Bill Marsden. Otherwise, it would be kind of a borderline story for us." He sighed. "Because we'll need to put in a lot of work on this. Oh, well. Screw the firemen. I guess Africa's nearer Boston than New York."

I said, "What does that mean?"

He smiled. "I'm sorry," he said. "I guess I should explain. My job is to oversee the output of thirteen newspapers, three TV stations, and a raft of radio stations. Mr. Poliakoff's job is to make money for the shareholders of the corporation of which the newspapers and radio and TV stations make up a small part. I'm a journalist first, a businessman second. Mr. Poliakoff's priorities are . . . the other way about." For a second, the lines around his eyes made him look tired. "So we have to sell things to Mr. Poliakoff . . . a certain way."

His neat face was alive again. There was an infectious warmth in his voice. He was an easy man to like.

"Hang in there," he said.

The door opened. A voice said, "Who wants me?"

It was a deep voice, with a chesty crunch like a punt's keel running onto shingle. It hauled itself out of the barrel chest of a man in a loose Savile Row pinstripe suit, standing in the deep carpet with his feet planted wide apart, knees slightly bent, as if the world were a small boat he had decided to keep level.

Pierce said, "George Devis, this is Serge Poliakoff."

Poliakoff had a handshake like an electric blanket. His eyes were gleaming chips of blue that came and went behind nets of folds and wrinkles in his big brown face. He said, "And what can we do for Mr. Devis?"

Ricky Lee was emanating the sureness of a hunter with the big bear in her sights. She said in an even, casual voice, "George is your next campaign, Mr. Poliakoff."

Poliakoff subjected her to the scrutiny of the chips of sapphire. He took note of her legs, her breasts, her slanted eyes. It was a powerful man's inventory. It should have been insulting, but instead it was impersonal. *Can I use this? What's it worth?* "Who are you?" he said.

Pierce stepped in. "Serge, this is Ricky Lee Klaasen. Miss Klaasen's a reporter attached to the Boston *Echo*." He made it sound as if they had been friends for years.

"Good," said Poliakoff. His lips were rubbery as he smiled. The eyes ceased inventorizing. "So tell me a story."

Ricky Lee told him the story. She told it well, except that I came out unnecessarily heroic. Poliakoff nodded, as if she were confirming things he already knew.

"So," said Poliakoff to me, when she had finished. "You're a sailor."

"An amateur."

Poliakoff grinned. "Two-handed across the Atlantic, and he's an amateur. I love it." He cast himself into an armchair and frowned at his knee. "But an experienced amateur. I seem to remember that you used to race with Martin Devereux."

I stared at him. Devereux was a neighbor in Pulteney, who had been one of the top ten match racers in the world before he had married an American and taken over a boatyard. I had helped him race a season when I was eighteen. We had come within an inch of qualifying for the Captain's Cup; even so, that had been an easy ten years ago. I said, "Clever of you to remember."

He smiled the rubbery smile. "It is the important things you remember," he said. "Lesser things I can leave to my research department." He picked up a telephone and made some calls. When he had finished, he said, "Mr. Devis, I'd like to help you. Let me explain some things."

He put up a thick brown hand, ticked off his forefinger. "One, we have espoused a lot of charitable causes, as a matter of corporate policy. Myself, I came from your Navy in the war. I was in Europe, a disaster area. Your Navy took me and . . . molded me, taught me techniques I could use to put my wishes into effect. This taught me the value of a push in the right direction. It is my duty to use this power to help my fellow man, my shareholders, myself." He grinned his pirate grin. "Not necessarily in that order."

He ticked off another finger. "Two, I had a great respect for Bill Marsden as a reporter, and for Rhydian Walters, as a singer and of course a . . . folk hero. I am sorry to say I never knew your sister." He said it with the kind of sincerity that made you believe it was a surprise to him to discover there was somebody in the world he had not met. "We must continue to explore what happened to these people. I think that if we have a campaign with you at the center, we may be able to . . . draw out some facts." He folded his hands over the waistcoat of his enormous suit. "But there is something," he said. "This is a tough, high-profile campaign we are talking about. How do I know you are a fit man to be its focus?"

Rapaport said, "I don't think there'll be a problem. Mr. Devis has sailed across the Atlantic. Ricky Lee assures me he's an excellent public speaker."

Poliakoff's eyes rested on me. Their glitter was the automatic glitter of stone. "Yes," he said. "But they tell me you write poems and books about birds. This campaign will not be about hearts and flowers. What I need to know is, are you a fighter, Mr. Devis?"

I said, "Who do you want me to fight?"

The eyes were heavy, ruminative. "I tell you what," he said. The smile came back; wide, rubber-lipped, carnivorous. "You used to race little boats. We'll take you up to Marblehead."

I gazed right back at him. Ricky Lee was sitting bolt upright, radiating anxiety. I found myself not liking Mr. Poliakoff. I said, "What happens in Marblehead?"

He said, "Tomorrow is Saturday. My playing day. I think we should go sailing."

"Sailing?"

"We will have a little race. You will need a crew. Shall we meet here at six o'clock tomorrow morning?"

I looked at his wide face. I sniffed the perfumed air, in which there now seemed to be a sharper note.

He said, "I believe you are interested in a Ras Hamil."

My heart thudded in my chest. I said, "That's right."

He smiled. He said, "I greatly look forward to our race, Mr. Devis. Until tomorrow, then." The hand enfolded mine, and he was gone.

I said, "What the hell was that about?"

Pierce Rapaport's aristocratic features were veiled with embarrassment. "Moxie test," he said. "If it's any consolation, he did it to me, too."

"And what happens?"

"You let him win, by a little."

"And then?"

Pierce smiled. "You have the power of PKC behind you. TV stations. Radio stations. And a worldwide industrial base: manufacturing, mining, oil. Contributing profits and information. Ras Hamil killed your sister and her husband, I believe? Well, Mr. Poliakoff has companies in Ethiopia." He smiled. "You'll just have to wait and see. Now. How about a crew?"

I said, "I'll dig someone up."

He said, "Good luck. They'll be expecting you at the Poliakoff Center. It's a hotel. See you tomorrow."

At the bottom of the gangway, Ricky Lee said, "We made it!"

I said, "Can you sail?"

She shook her head.

I said, "I'll call you tomorrow." My head was in the village. In the heat, and the smell of ashes, and the terror. All the way over here in America, this man Poliakoff knows about Ras Hamil. This powerful man. Thanks to Ricky Lee. I said, "Thank you very much."

She winked. I gave her a ride downtown. She disappeared into Boston.

I drove to the Poliakoff Center, and called Rooney's in Quogue. Danny Rooney answered. I said, "Can you get a message to Scotch John?"

Danny said, "I'll send Festus out."

"Tell him to find a car and get himself down here. We're racing tomorrow, six A.M." I left the number and went to my room.

I got a telephone call from the switchboard at ten o'clock. John had arrived and was waiting in the bar. I went down.

He was sitting on a stool like a black bear that had strayed into a drawing room. There was a half-empty beer glass at his elbow, and his hands were moving over the lanyard he was knotting.

He said, "What's this race?"

I told him about Poliakoff.

He nodded. He said, "I heard of this guy. Friendship sloops, he sails. Outta Marblehead, God knows why."

I said, "What's a Friendship sloop?"

"Fast boat," he said. "Used to be a workboat, out of Friendship, up Muscongus Bay. They ain't a sloop. More like a cutter. Three foresails, gaff topsail. Who's crewing?"

"You and me."

His heavy black eyebrows went up. His teeth appeared in his beard. "How many's Poliakoff got?"

"I don't know."

"Five, I guess," he said. "Forgive me asking, but why are we racing?"

I said, "I came to America to raise money to carry on the work my sister and Rhyd were doing in Africa. If we do okay in this race, Poliakoff will help out."

He gazed at me. "Do okay?"

I ordered a beer. I said, "Someone said I ought to let Mr. Poliakoff win."

John folded away his sinnet. "That's what you want to do, you do it," he said. Behind the beard, his face was impenetrable. "I gotta catch some zees."

I went to bed myself. I lay there, twenty-one floors above downtown Boston, and thought about the favor I had found with Mr. Poliakoff. I thought of the advantages to PloughShare of a well-publicized lecture tour. I thought of the advantages to me of the research facilities of a big organization like Poliakoff Communications, with particular regard to Ras Hamil.

But most of all, I thought about Rhyd and Camilla, and what they would have thought of fat cats like Poliakoff. I had been a coward once, and I did not like the idea of being one again. I knew that none of us would have liked the idea of letting him win.

And whatever Pierce said, I did not see Poliakoff as a man who would be impressed by a loser.

11

*A*T FIVE-THIRTY THE NEXT MORNING, THE STREETS OF BOSTON were mostly empty. There were a few joggers, the odd dog walker. The sky was blue. As I drove Scotch John toward the docks, the steam from the stacks on the high-rise banks had only the faintest downwind curve.

The matelot at the foot of the gangplank raised an eyebrow at the Mustang and showed me a garage in one of the big, dirty blocks facing on to the quay. John looked over the *Duchess* with admiration, but without awe. We walked up the gangway at one minute to six. There was a breakfast table laid for ten in the dining saloon: white cloth, silver knives and forks, silver chafing dishes with domed lids. Pierce was waiting for us with four men. They were big men, dark brown, wearing blue blazers and white duck trousers and beautiful new Docksiders. John was wearing a Grateful Dead T-shirt, Levis and his samosa deck shoes. Pierce introduced us. The big men had teeth as white as their trousers, handshakes like giant lobsters, and absolutely no tattoos. The largest was called Craig Bigelow. I had seen him in the racing pages of several yachting magazines. He said, "I saw you had a problem in the Transatlantic."

"That's right," I said. He wanted me to think about problems. "You sail yourself?"

One of his crew tittered. Pierce was standing behind them. He winked at me. He said, "Craig is skipper of *Tempest*, Mr. Poliakoff's maxi."

"Nice boat," said John. "Leastways, will be when someone tunes the sucker right."

There was a pale, horrid silence. *Tempest* was an eighty-foot bobsleigh which regularly raced on one of the world's most skillful and expensive circuits. Last season, there had been a lot of seconds and thirds, but no wins. Craig and his crew would not like the implication that their boat was under-tuned.

Pierce caught my eye. He looked amused. He said, "How's about some breakfast, everybody?"

As we sat down, a faint tremor of engines came through the deck and the dockside warehouses started to slide past the big windows. John pulled a couple of silver chafing dishes toward him and shoveled sausages and pancakes on to his plate. He then walked around the table, appropriated some eggs and bacon, and said to a white-coated steward, "Can I get some syrup?"

The syrup arrived. He hosed down the pyramid of food with it, shoveled half a pound into his mouth, chewed noisily. When he had half finished the mouthful, he said to the steward, "Can I get a beer?"

There was a frightful silence. Bigelow took an ostentatious sip of orange juice. The beer arrived. So did Serge Poliakoff, big as a barn in a double-breasted blazer with Royal Flotilla buttons. "Morning," he said. "Sorry I'm late." He smiled. There were papery bags of skin under his eyes. He looked as if he could have been up all night. "Beer all right? One of my airlines flies it in from the brewery."

John said, "Sure," belched, and pronged another sausage. The silence intensified.

"Very good," said Poliakoff, watching him. "Now maybe I should explain. This is a little bit of fun for me, this race. We'll motor up to Marblehead. There in half an hour. I've got a couple of nice little boats up there. Identical. We'll sail. That all the crew you've got?"

I said, "That's all." I was watching him, biding my time, a flutter of excitement in the stomach.

He smiled the big, rubber-lipped smile. The eyes had a new glitter. Mr. Poliakoff was excited, too. "On your own head be it," he said. "Two-handed is okay transatlantic. Here . . . well."

Craig's eyes were small and blue and mean. He said, "I heard you sank." He was still trying to get my mind on to trouble.

I said, "That's right." I sipped coffee.

"And they never found the guy who did it."

"That's right," I said.

"You were lying last in the race, right?" he said. "You sure it was someone? Wasn't just the boat fell apart?"

Poliakoff was watching closely. "Machine guns first," I said. "Then they rammed us."

Craig's mouth twitched up at the corners. "Yeah," he said. "Happens all the time. What'd you been smoking?"

His crew laughed. Poliakoff drank coffee.

The palms of my hands were wet with anger. Blow the psychology, I thought. I have got to beat this man.

More coffee came in, and Scotch John drank another beer. Poliakoff unfolded a chart of Marblehead on the table. There were three buoys in a long, thin triangle. Outside the windows the sea slid past flat and blue, ruffled with breeze now. There was a faint silvering at the eastern margins of the world, as if there was fog waiting out there.

"Rules," said Poliakoff. "Twice around. Standard match. Neutral judge on the water."

I said, "Who's that?"

"Claud Bowler," he said. "Very nice guy." He paused. The grin was big enough to show gold molars. "Anglophile."

After breakfast, we went on deck. The *Duchess of Malfi* was loping across the water with the ponderous force of a cantering draft horse. Ahead was a rocky bay and a sprawl of timber buildings. "Rich guys' heaven," said John.

The *Duchess* slid past an island and came alongside a timber staging. There were more yachts ahead of us. The *Duchess's* space was clear. As the matelots jumped about with the mooring warps, I found myself yawning. I looked at my watch. It was not yet ten past seven in the morning.

Poliakoff lit a fresh cigar. "Well, gentlemen," rumbled the big voice. "You want to look at a boat? Race starts eight-fifteen."

"Sure," I said.

Win the race. Raise the money. *In the name of your sister, and of God.*

We walked down the gangway. The dock's planks were smooth and unsplintered. There were damp patches that might have been an overnight shower, or someone up early scrubbing gullshit. Craig Bigelow and his gorillas padded on ahead in their matching deck shoes. Poliakoff waved his cigar at the houses. "Nice place," he said. "Seventeenth century, some of these. Quiet. Can't stand the noise. Peace. Seclusion."

"Costs a lot," said John, coming straight to the point.

"An awful lot," said Poliakoff, who had no genteel scruples about talking money. "But we look after it, so it gets to be worth more."

We stopped on the quay above two pretty, snipe-beaked yachts. They had big, long cockpits and slender bowsprits. Their fidded topmasts gave them a quaint, archaic air. They gleamed with varnish, and their brasswork shone buttery yellow.

"Someone bin polishin' these," said John.

"Like I said," said Poliakoff. "We look after them, so they get worth more. You sure you can manage, just the two of you?"

There were three forestays, which meant three headsails. There was a gaff topsail. It was a tall mast. It looked as if it would be an easy mast to lose over the side. I said, "Sure I can manage. How many are you carrying?"

Poliakoff said, "Five." He was grinning.

I said, "Bullshit."

Poliakoff's eyes turned wary. He said, "What do you suggest?"

"Crew of two per boat."

Poliakoff said, "No. I insist." I realized he had expected I would cave in. I thought, surprised: This man seriously wants to win, and will cheat to do it.

A small man in a peaked cap was walking along the quay. He had a genuine nautical roll and a face that looked like sandblasted leather. He said, "Howdy, Mr. Poliakoff."

Poliakoff swiveled his eyes on him. His face stiffened. He said, "Morning, Claud. You ready?"

Claud said, "What we got?"

Poliakoff introduced us.

"Hmm," said Claud. He had old yellowish eyes that knew more than they gave away. "That was you went down on the Early Atlantic Race? Bad stuff."

I agreed it was bad stuff.

"Just the two again?" said Claud. "Lot of strings on them Friendships. But they sail real sweet."

Poliakoff's bright eyes moved between me and Claud. He detected a sympathy between us—he had excellent antennae. I sensed that Claud's approval mattered to him almost as much as winning races. I also sensed that Claud found Poliakoff an influential friend and patron. Poliakoff nodded to himself, said, "And I'll take Mr. Bigelow and David. I'll be sailing as owner and observer."

"Sounds fair," said Claud. "Tough morning's work for all. Thank Christ I'm too old for anything but engines."

Round one, even Stephen. Three against two.

We walked across to the outside boat. Poliakoff and his two crew stayed on the inside.

We took off the sail covers and hoisted a staystail. John cast off. The wind peeled the nose off the quay. As we slid toward the harbor entrance, he pulled up the rest of the sails. He said, "Watch the staysail."

The quay end went by surprisingly fast. The boom was long, the gaff peak high. Forward of the mast were three sails, one at the end of the bowsprit, the second on the forestay, the third a little triangle of white canvas flying like a kite high up by the button on the top of the topmast. I moved the nose up toward the wind. The staysail fluttered as the breeze tickled the wrong side of the luff. The deck lifted, uncertain under my deck shoes as the aerofoil deformed and the power faltered. When I glanced over my shoulder I saw another tower of sail moving the other side of the breakwater. The other Friendship slid out from behind the quay like a lunging plesiosaur. Her staysail was out of control, drumming and roaring. Her gaff mainsail looked flat and shapeless. Claud followed in a semirigid inflatable.

John said, "He hasn't got the people he's used to."

Craig was at the tiller. A blue cloud of smoke whisked across the green water from Poliakoff's cigar. I guessed that Claud's eyesight was none too good. "Watch him," I said. "He may join in."

We had forty minutes for practice. I would have preferred a week. We did the best we could. I took her out to a chunk of clear air and tried her on various points of sail. Like a lot of gaff-rigged boats, she was very fast on a broad reach. To windward, clawing her way zigzag into the eye of the breeze, she was slower, because going to windward is a matter of tuning the soft aerofoils of the sails, and an old gaff-rigged boat has a lot of slots and spars to interfere with the laminar flow of wind over curved cloth.

But John had sailed Friendships before. He looked as if he had sailed them well. And a two-handed transatlantic race is good practice for running a complicated boat short-handed.

Craig might be a world-class hired gun, but he was a hired gun who was used to racing with a crew of twenty serious athletes.

I looked at my watch. Ten minutes to start time. The *Duchess of Malfi* had moved out of the bay and was hovering like a miniature liner on the gray-green chop. Between us and her was a squat red can buoy. Together, they marked the two ends of the start line.

John said, "He's coming into the area."

The area is an imaginary triangle behind the start line, which serves as an arena for the gladiators taking part in a two-boat race. The other boat was powering in, silver foam roaring from her cutwater, her sails a mountain of white in the sun.

John said, "She looks real pretty, all that varnish and all."

He was right. The other Friendship looked as if it had just sailed out of a broker's advertisement. The sun struck brilliant highlights from the brass of a porthole. I thought of what Poliakoff had said about things getting more valuable when carefully looked after. He was a man attached to inanimate objects, particularly when they represented money. I said, "It would be dreadful to bend it."

John coughed. "Dreadful," he said.

A puff of wind grayed the green on the port bow. I eased the tiller as the Friendship heeled, dug in her lee rail, pulling white plumes of water off her stanchions. We were going fast now, the wake sluicing away like a salmon river. Now it was just our boat, and the other boat, and the wind, and the line.

I told John what I wanted to do.

He pulled his beard. "No problem," he said. "Unless the other guy knows more'n we do."

"Hope for the best," I said.

He let off the mainsheet, waited. We slowed, jilling along, sails flapping up a thunder in the blue morning sky.

"Now," he said, and hauled in the mainsheet.

She began to move.

The wake moved from a gurgle to a bubble, from a bubble to a roar. The stanchions went back in and the white water hissed like a basket of snakes. The cloud of canvas became rigid, powered up with forty kilowatts of breeze. The hull tilted until the overhangs leaned confidentially into the water.

She moved like a torpedo, her bowsprit pointing well ahead

of the bowsprit on the other boat. If I kept this course, there was a chance I could squeak under the charging ram of his bowsprit, tack ahead of him, steal his wind.

Just a chance.

I saw Bigelow's face a hundred and fifty yards away, squinting at me over a hand-bearing compass. A puff of wind bore the mast over to starboard, laying her steeply on her side. Water sloshed into the cockpit, filling my shoes. I luffed, pulling the nose further ahead. Those bastards are aiming to pass under my nose, he would be thinking. I am on starboard tack, with right-of-way. He would be beginning to feel confident.

Because we were not going to make it.

12

OUR BOWSPRIT WAS STILL POINTING AHEAD OF HIS. BUT HE WOULD have taken his bearings and watched the distance the wind was blowing us sideways, and he would be grinning.

I kept on, the tiller jumping a little under my hand as it caught the eddies from the long, slippery hull. If I crashed into him, we would be disqualified.

We would also bend Serge Poliakoff's beautiful antique boat, with Craig at the helm, under the owner's nose. It would be my fault. But it would be a big psychological problem for Craig.

They were all looking now. I luffed, aiming the nose too high into the wind, trying to look as if I was pinching to get in front of his bowsprit. The sails bellied and thundered, and the run of the hull weakened underfoot. I said, "Here we go."

The side of the other Friendship was fifty feet away. Forty. Thirty. There was no time to tack now. I was going to hit him halfway down his length, the classic T-bone. There was a lot of roaring going on, and not only of canvas. I tried to look shocked and horrified, a man who had misjudged, out of his depth in a strange boat. It was not difficult. I held my course, watching his sails.

I saw what I had been looking for.

Up there in the sky, his staysail shivered. Then his topsail went, and the luff of the main.

He was putting on the brakes; not because he was certain of a collision, but because he was worried about bending the boat.

Our bowsprit was ten feet from his side when I hauled the tiller toward me. Water roared over the rudder. The bowsprit swept his afterdeck, but touched nothing. We shot under his stern.

"Tacking," I said, and shoved the tiller away from me.

John ran up the side deck. The three foresails clapped a couple of times, came hard in. When I looked under the boom, the other boat was dead in the water, everything flapping, and someone was yelling at someone to back a foresail to bring her around.

Craig's face was the color of raw liver. Claud Bowler was leaning back in the seat of his inflatable, shrugging, spreading his hands, laughing. There is no rule against bluffing someone to a standstill.

"Ten seconds till the gun," said John.

Thirty-five seconds after the gun, we waltzed over the line five boat lengths ahead. We held the lead twice around the course.

"Lawdy, lawdy," said John, as we crossed the line. "I thought this Bigelow was supposed to know something."

I said, "He was being careful of the boss's boat."

John said, "He didn't throw nothing at us."

I was feeling terrific. The sun was out, it was ten A.M. and we had won. I took the boat back, and came alongside under sail.

A shadow darkened the silvery timbers of the deck. I looked up. Poliakoff was standing over us, a mountainous black silhouette against the morning sun. "Devis, you're a bastard," he said. His rumbling voice was shaking. I realized he was laughing. "Do you know what, Devis? I rather like a bastard. I actually rather do. Bloody impressive. But you'll have to be kind to poor Craig now. When you're ready, come back to the *Duchess*."

The tender took us out. Craig sat as far away as possible. We reported to the cabin with silk walls. Poliakoff shot the cork of a bottle of pink Krug at the wall next to a Van de Velde and filled the glasses. He raised his glass, his eyes bright blue cracks above the rubbery slot of teeth. He walked across to me and said, "You've proved your point. Pierce is on board somewhere. He'll take you where you need to be. I'll brief him."

I found I was looking into the stony blue eyes. I said, "What about Ras Hamil?"

He smiled. He said, "Wait and see, Mr. Devis."

He touched his glass with his lips; put it down. "Excuse me." He left the cabin.

A couple of minutes later Pierce came in. He said to me, "I need you this morning."

"When?"

"Soon as we dock. George Devis is going to become a public figure."

I said, "One thing. Why did you tell me to throw the race?"

Pierce grinned. He said, "We have no time for people who can stand to lose."

The *Duchess* came alongside. White-bloused matelots scurried about with warps and springs. There was a black limousine between the bollards. "That's us," he said. "Let's go."

I offered the Mustang keys to John. He refused. "See you in Quogue," he said. Pierce drove me to a studio. They interviewed me for thirty minutes, and edited it down to three minutes of the six o'clock news hour.

I thought I knew about TV, because of the Anglia natural history films. This bore no resemblance to natural history. The anchorman extracted the story with the precision of a master of wine's corkscrew. What came out had nothing to do with the slow, plodding process of foreign aid, PloughShare style. It was an epic of linked murders salted with the hellish randomness of fate. Bill Marsden turned out to have been one of the East Coast's best-loved investigative journalists. I turned out to be a reclusive genius, combining the best points of Christopher

Columbus, Charles Audubon and Alexander Pope. They talked a lot about Rhyd and Camilla and PloughShare, but cut the stuff about Ras Hamil. "Too much at one time," they said. "This one will run. Think of it as a serial."

Pierce met me outside the studio. "Brilliant." He seemed to be talking about me. "So don't believe me," he said. "Believe the people. We have seventy-two thousand dollars in pledges. The phones are still going. Come up to the office. I'll run the tape."

We went up to a big office with two forty-inch screens.

There was me, talking about sudden death, looking stringy and bronzed and British. Then there was a handful of starvation statistics, Rhyd playing "The Alleluia Tree" on the Country Cousins world hookup, pictures of Poliakoff standing in front of a pallet of grain bags under a banner screaming BOSTON ECHO DASH TO AFRICA. "That was the last campaign," said Pierce. "Mozambique. Serge can't stay out of it." One of his eyebrows was a millimeter higher than the other. I got the feeling that working for Poliakoff could be a strain. There was a good final plug from the anchorman. Pierce poured me a glass of whiskey. I drank it so quickly I hardly noticed it was there. He poured more.

I said, "How well did you know Bill Marsden?"

He said, "I don't have too much direct contact with news any more." He looked faintly rueful. "Usual story, I'm afraid. You get good at something, they stop you doing it."

I rang Jerry Stein at the PloughShare office in Bristol. I said, "It seems to be working."

Jerry said, "I'm delighted. For us. For you, too."

I knew what he meant. For the first time in months, the shame had gone to the back of my mind.

Another telephone rang. Pierce answered it. His eyebrows went up. He said, "Mr. Diglis, he's right here." He passed me the receiver.

The voice on the other end was smooth and deep and dark. It said, "Hello, George."

"Who's this?"

"Warren Diglis here. George, I think you should stop this campaign."

I said, "Do you really?"

"There are a lot of us out here who do not like your neocolonialist bullshit, George. We know that when you picking up charity money, you got glue on your hands. So we want you to stop this, and leave it to us who knows. We have a black solution to a black problem, George. You stay away."

I said, "I don't know what you're talking about."

He said, "Stay away," and laughed a smooth, dark, cold laugh. The line went dead.

I put the receiver down.

Pierce said, "Warren tell you it's not your problem?"

"That's right." I sipped whiskey. I was too excited by all the rest of it to be brought down by a voice on the end of a telephone. "Who is he?"

"Fight manager. Conscience of black America, self-appointed. Did a stretch for armed robbery in his youth, made himself over. Lot of influential friends, particularly friends who need black votes." Pierce sat for a moment looking at his softly gleaming shoes. Ivy League and impenetrable. "Pay no attention," he said. He raised his eyes. "I wonder, can I make a suggestion?"

"Suggestion?"

He poured more whiskey. He said, "Impertinence, really. Put this down as an out-to-grass editor tinkering. But I spoke to Ricky Lee about these lectures of yours. She's inexperienced, but there's an . . . acuteness about her. When you're speaking now, at these lunches, I think you ought to make it personal. Move in on Ras Hamil. But can you find some kind of focus beyond that? Ricky Lee tells me it was kind of diffuse." He dropped his eyes, embarrassed. "You're a poet, right? You've read poetry aloud, I know. I hate to tell you what to do. But there's a . . . well, a coldness to a straight lecture. Try to think of this as a low-rent poetry reading. You're at the Cambridge

Regency tomorrow. You should have a real sympathetic crowd. Is there some way you can dig out a single image you can hang it all on?"

I thought: Devis, they are screwing with the content. But these were the people who had made seventy thousand dollars for PloughShare. They were trained to screw with the content. If they wanted me to hang images on something, I would ransack the joint for hooks.

I said, "There's the Alleluia Tree."

"Wow," he said. "What's that?"

I told him.

"Ras Hamil," he said. "We can start picking up on that. The man who burned the Alleluia Tree. George, I think we have a winner."

I drove him in the Mustang to a restaurant given over to oak paneling and lobsters. His wife joined us. She was dark and pretty and she had read my poetry. It was a good evening, more like dinner with friends than with business acquaintances. At the end, Pierce said, "I'm glad Ricky Lee brought you in. It's nice to get a chance to do something that's useful to someone besides the shareholders."

We shook hands.

"See you at lunch tomorrow," he said.

I went back to my room at the Poliakoff Center and started on the speech. The fear was gone. Now I had power, and PloughShare was getting money. The things I should have made happen in the village were happening in Boston.

Lunch the next day was not recognizable as the same meal as the one swallowed in the house of Mrs. Portarlington Elliott. Poliakoff's TV and radio stations had been yelling about it since the previous night. The story of Bill's murder was in the geometric center of the front page of the newspaper room service brought me. I went and looked at George Devis, international hero, in the mirror. I had finished working on the speech at four A.M. The face was gaunter than usual. There were black circles under the eyes, echoing the soreness in the head started by one too many glasses of Quincy at dinner and hammered home by the Poliakoff Center's air conditioning. I parked the Mustang down from the Cambridge Regency where the lunch was being held. There were policemen holding back the crowds, and four television crews. There was even a small demonstration, with placards bearing the legend THE SUN ALREADY SET ON THE BRITISH EMPIRE. Pierce was waiting, looking like a particularly intelligent hawk in a charcoal gray suit. He introduced me to a couple of senators. We all grinned for the photographers. We ate rubber chicken. I told the story of Ras Hamil and the Alleluia Tree, plain and simple. People wept. At the end, the donations totaled forty-one thousand dollars. Someone from the Boston *Echo* collected the checks. They even had a credit card machine.

Pierce went off to his next meeting. When the handshaking stopped, Ricky Lee came out of the crowd and tucked her hand under my arm. She said, "Isn't that all worthwhile?"

I grinned at her. I said, "I am truly and sincerely grateful."

She smiled at me from her wonky eyes. She said, "You did me a favor, too. I guess we all win. Listen, I can't find Sullivan."

"Sullivan?"

"The editor. I'm still looking. I have to go interview someone."

"I'll be in Quogue." I gave her the number of Rooney's.

She said, "See you. Thanks again, right?"

I watched her go, her cheerful, elegant strut pulling politically incorrect eyes after her as she went through the crowd in the lobby.

A voice said, "A word."

I looked around. The voice belonged to a wide man with a face the color of milky coffee and a saddle of darker spots across the bridge of a nose that had at some time in his life been hit by something ugly and hard, like a prison sentence. The eyes were big, but narrow. The hair was frizzy and gray.

The mouth opened. The eyes did not. The man said, "Stop this, right now."

The face was the face of a fighter. After a lunch like this one, fighters did not bother me. I said, "Stop what?"

"This speechifying," he said. "You ripping us off." The voice was deep, dark and cold. I had heard it before, on the telephone at the TV station.

"Ripping who off?"

"My name is Warren Diglis," he said. "I am a personal friend of Mr. Ras Hamil."

I looked into his narrow black eyes. I thought of machine guns. I said, "Your personal friend destroyed my family."

He said, "You can prove that?"

I said, "Of course." I thought of Mr. Gugsa with the skullcap of curly hair, of the crowd in the clay street of the village. My mind began to shrivel as I caught the whiff of bitter ashes and terror.

He said, "I don't believe you can. Because it ain't true." He smiled. It was a cold, crocodilian smile. He said, "Now you look after yourself, you hear?" He fixed me with the cold eyes. They seemed to burrow into my head, looking for the seat of terror. He walked away.

The crowd had gone. The euphoria congealed. My footsteps rang on the high concrete buildings as I walked down the sidewalk to the meter where I had left the car. The street was long and gray, receding to a hazy vanishing point three blocks away. I took the key out of my pocket to open the driver's door. I stopped.

Someone had caved in the rear window of the passenger side nearest the pavement. There was glass all over the back seat. When I walked around the back end, I saw the edge of the boot was bent and cracked. The lid came up easily when I hooked my finger under it. My bag was still there, but someone had unpacked it messily. A pair of almost new Docksiders was gone, and so was the spare wheel. They had left the clothes.

I stood there and swore in a gentle, personal manner.

Someone cleared his throat at my elbow. I looked down. There was a very small fat man with ears that stuck out like cup handles below a Florida Vacationland baseball cap. "Robbed," he said. The super king-size cigarette in the center of his mouth jiggled as he talked. His voice was high and he smelled of old tobacco. "I seen 'em."

My heart was hammering in my chest. I said, "They pinched my shoes."

"Yeah," said the fat man. "And your spare. Ain't nothing safe in this town. I sell papers." He pointed at a sort of kiosk on the corner. "I seen it all."

"Who was it?"

"One white one. One black boy," said the fat midget. "Druggers, I guess."

I thanked him, extricated myself from his clutches, repacked the suitcase, and called the police, who said more or less the same thing and were not at all interested. I bought some more shoes, and found an artist's supply shop, where I picked up some gouache and watercolors, and half a dozen blocks of heavy handmade paper. Then, with no reluctance at all, I drove my pounding head out of town and up the coast.

It is about four hours' driving from Boston to Quogue. After a while, I stopped being angry about the car. I turned off the highway, wound through the pines and rock outcrops to Quogue, and parked the car outside Rooney's.

Danny turned his pasty face upon me. He said, "Scotch John come?"

I thanked him for delivering the message. "Any letters?" I asked.

He shook his head. "No calls, neither. John come home this morning. He'll be on the boat."

The smile on my face felt frozen with disappointment. I had not realized exactly how much I was worrying about the boys. I thought: Give them a couple more days. I bought some cans of Budweiser to go and walked back onto the quay.

There was fog hovering out there. Beyond the lobster boats, the black trees of Quogue Island floated on a silver cushion. I took the Mustang up to Ray's AutoBody, and walked back down to the quay with my bag.

A scaup drifted across the gray glass of the harbor, towing a line of ducklings like a tug towing coal tubs. I searched along the dinghies moored to the quay until I found where I had moored the one that said *Tender to Halcyon*. It was a timber dory, a miniature version of the ones the schooners used to drop to jig for cod on the Grand Banks. A typical Rhyd boat: not beautiful, but sturdy and workmanlike. A good tool.

I rowed out toward the moorings in the center of the blue gray disk of the water. On the boat I popped a beer and slung my bag down the hatch. The lecture schedule said I was due in Rochester, New Hampshire, the day after tomorrow. I was worried about the boys. I was worried about Warren Diglis. I do not like being worried when there is nothing I can do about it.

The sun was drifting down into the fog, tinging the gray pink, like blood in water. I went below, lit the stove. I pulled out a watercolor block and a brush and washed it gray, with an edge for the black rim of Quogue Rock. Somewhere out in the fog, a loon let rip with a long, despairing yodel. I put in the trees, laid the pink on the fog. Ripples clocked. The scaup hustled by, towing her chicks, sharp against the sun as if they were cut out of black paper. I painted them in.

Painting had always been a good way of calming the uncertainties of life. Perhaps that was why it had been incompatible with Mary Morpurgo, who liked to cultivate rather than calm uncertainties. She and I had lived together for a year and a bit, during which I had accompanied her on five poetry tours and she had come sailing for three weeks. She had been on a sixth tour when I had sailed *Auk* around to Essex, picked her up from Maldon quay after she had been reading at the Poly, and shanghaied her out into the Thames Estuary.

It had been July, one of those nights when it seems not to get fully dark. *Auk* had sat there at anchor in the gurgle of the tide. Mary had gone to bed early. I had stayed up late, watching the full moon, feeling the tug of it as it towed the heavy sheet of dirty water up the throat of the North Sea. I had dozed, and at dawn pulled out the paintbox. The light was wash-gray and butter-yellow over the swales and mudbanks. The sun and moon hung in the sky at opposite sides of the world, as if on the same huge, invisible seesaw. Inside this matrix of forces, scribbles of duck and geese wrote messages on the sky and the water. I painted for an hour. Then Mary came on deck, naked as a practicing witch.

"God," she said. "Doesn't that mud *stink?* Can we go ashore? This is so *boring.*"

Two weeks afterward, she disappeared to Barcelona with a performance poet. I missed her. But not as much as I would have missed painting if someone had told me it had to stop.

Tonight in Quogue, it took me four tries at the scaup before I got her right.

The engine of the dusk was starting up. The birds were driving it: *Here we are,* they were yelling. *Keep off. I love you. I'm hungry.* There were gulls in it, waders, duck, divers. The sun slid into the fog. I forgot to paint. I sat there and listened.

The night was getting cold. I went below. The saloon was warming up. I found a clothes peg, hung the painting to dry, fried some eggs and bacon. Then I spread a sleeping bag on the starboard berth, climbed in and went out like a light.

Next morning, the sky was blue through the portholes and lobster-boat engines rattled in the calm. I made a cup of coffee, picked up the sketch pad and clambered into the cockpit. To seaward, John's houseboat was hanging off a mooring buoy made of a bundle of tires and oil drums. The upperworks had been extended with a series of galleries and shanties, from which stovepipes and aerials bristled like the spines of a porcupine. John was on the topmost gallery, dragging a sheet of corrugated iron. He waved. The blows of his hammer floated across the water. I drank some coffee and ate a stale bagel. I painted a quick sketch of the harbor for the boys, marking *Halcyon's* mooring with an X. Then I rowed over to John's boat.

It might once have been a tug. He had converted the aft side of the bridge into a veranda and there was a Ping-Pong table where the towline horse had once been.

I skirted a crowd of bastard ducks milling around the straw-covered pontoon on the port side, climbed over the rail and tied up to a bollard between two fifty-gallon drums in which potato plants were growing. There was a bell with a round sinnet pull. I pulled it.

A door opened. John's head appeared. "Hi," he said. "Come in."

Once, it had been the crew's quarters. Now, most of the walls were covered in ornamental ropework. There was stained glass in the portholes and a strong smell of marijuana in the air. A stereo was issuing lazy flatpicked guitar; then Rhyd's voice, double-tracked, high harmony a third above the tune: *Teaching you sense is like digging a hole in a lake.*

John made coffee. I said, "I wanted to thank you for coming to Boston."

"Pleasure," he said. "Always nice to sail a Friendship." He grinned. "Always nice to win a race." He had pulled out some string and was starting another series of knots. "But you ain't here just for the racing."

I told him about the lecture tour. He nodded. There was a glassiness to his eyes. We sat in silence. The tape auto-reversed. Rhyd kept on singing. Eventually, he said, "Who was it killed your sister and Rhyd?"

"Man called Ras Hamil," I said.

He raised his eyebrows. "Ah," he said. There was another silence. "Why did he do it?"

I said, "I don't know."

John said, "You interested to find out?"

I said, "Of course."

John said, "If ever you need help, you ask."

I said, "Fine."

He was looking at a framed photograph on the wall. There was a boat, a steel-hulled cutter, tied up alongside a quay. In the background were sheds and a dusty-looking palm tree. John was sitting on the cabin top. On one side of him was Rhyd, squinting against the sun. On the other side was a black woman in a white singlet.

He saw I was looking at the photograph. He nodded. *"Simoom,"* he said. "Out in Port Sudan, on the Red Sea. Used to take charter guys out diving. I was a big diver, then."

"When?"

"Last year. I went down to Port Sudan four years ago, right? Rhyd turns up a couple of years ago, charters me out for a little diving. We got pretty friendly, him and Camilla and me and Abeba. Abeba was the woman I was with at the time. Ol' Abeba. We used to go sailing, and we dived and I play this, well, *el primitivo* guitar, and we played some bars in Port Sudan, Egypt, up and down the coast, all kinds. We had a great time, last year, the year before. I guess he and Camilla were relaxing, really. Camilla said it was nice to see the ol' guy having a good time after the work he put in."

I could imagine Camilla saying it. She was always more interested in other people than in herself.

He picked up a packet of cigarette papers and a can of dope and rolled a joint. I do not like being around dopeheads. I left, rowed myself ashore.

There was still no letter from the boys.

I posted them my painting. Then I rang Ricky Lee, to see if she had found Sullivan. Ricky Lee was out. So I went back to the boat.

13

*N*EXT MORNING I PUT ON A SUIT AND ROWED ASHORE. THERE WAS still no mail from the boys. All right, I thought, that makes a week. Today, I visit. But first, I was on duty.

I picked up the Mustang from Ray's AutoBody and reported for duty in Rochester, New Hampshire, three-quarters of the way back to Boston. The lunch was in the house of a private citizen with no political connections that I knew of, so I did not expect a lot. Also, I was ready for a sense of anticlimax after the triumph at the Cambridge Regency.

But waiting in the house were sixty lunchers and a TV crew. The lunchers donated close to thirty thousand dollars. After the lady from the *Echo* had finished stuffing checks into envelopes and cranking the credit card machine, the TV crew did another interview, delving into precisely what Rhyd and Camilla had been doing in Ethiopia. The producer thanked me. He said, "You're right there on the six o'clock news again."

I said, "Is it that big a story?"

He pursed his lips and looked away. He said, "Forgive me. It ain't what you know, it's who you know."

"Mr. Poliakoff."

The producer grinned. He said, "Mr. Poliakoff's campaigns are great, when what he is using you for fits with what you want to do." He lit a cigarette. "So I get stories on to the six o'clock hour. And you get to be this fortnight's hero." A hero who had run away from the smell of ashes. He shook my hand. His palm was wet and nervous. "Thanks," he said.

I drove out of town, stopped at a garage and tried to call Ricky Lee. The answering service said she was out. Then I tried to call Sarah Ebden. There was no answer. I climbed back into the Mustang and drove east for Bethel Bay.

From the ridge where the track passed between the two hills I could see the pond, the black pines around the house and barns, the blue wedge of sea beyond. Among the barns, the windscreen of a pickup truck reflected a starburst of pale sun. I applied the foot gingerly to the accelerator and began to navigate my way through the potholes, craning my neck around for signs of Joe or Harry. There was something by the pond that was either a duck hunter's hide or an Ethiopian hut. Of actual boys there was no sign.

I slid the bonnet into the woods around the house, eyes probing the dapple of light and shade. I had missed the boys. I was excited at the prospect of seeing them again.

As I approached the gateway into the yard, a figure stepped into the pool of sunlight that lay across the road. It was Chuck. He was wearing a T-shirt and sawn-off brown canvas trousers. He stood in front of the car, immovable as a sandbag. His face looked bulging and sullen under the baseball cap. But I was not watching his face. I was watching his hands. In his hands he was holding his Mannlicher. The business end of the rifle was pointing straight into my left eye.

I said, "Good afternoon, Chuck."

His eyes were narrow and puffy. He said, "Git out that car."

My hands were suddenly slippery on the steering wheel. I said, "It's me. George Devis. The boys' uncle. Don't you remember me?"

A rope of saliva hung from his fat lower lip. "I don't remember nothin'," he said. "This is a security check. Git out."

This is bloody stupid, I thought. Except that there is nothing stupid about a rifle barrel in your left eye. "Where are the boys?" I said.

"Git out," he said.

I put my foot on the accelerator. The engine rumbled in its throat like a dog. I said, "Move, please."

He ran clumsily around the car. The only thing that was not clumsy was the round eye of the rifle, which stayed on me, steady as a rock. "Git out," he said. He jabbed the rifle through the open window and into my ear. It hurt like hell.

I said, "I wouldn't do that, if I were you."

Camilla's SAS man had shown me techniques by which I could have taken the rifle away from him and wrapped it around his neck. But he was my cousin by marriage, and he had a mental age of ten. It was also worth considering that he could blow my brains out with a twitch of the finger.

So I got out.

"English folks," said Chuck in a heavy voice, as if quoting from early-morning cartoons. "Who trusts 'em?"

I said, "When I tell your mother about you, she will not be happy."

Chuck said, "She said to be vig—to watch." He was playing guards. There would be no distinction in his mind between toy shells and live rounds.

I said, "Do we stand here all morning?"

A voice from the yard called, "Chuck!"

He screwed up his face, shook his head: Don't make a sound.

Suddenly, I felt happier. Chuck knew he was being a bad boy. "Here," I said.

Sarah came around the corner. She looked pale. Her hair had escaped its neat bun. It looked like the explosion of a blond-and-gray firework. I said, "Tell him to put that thing away."

She looked at me, then back at Chuck. She said, "Put it in the cabinet." Her voice was a long way away. So were her eyes. My heartbeat began to steady. Rhyd, I was thinking, why did you send your children here? Will or no will, this was a madhouse.

Chuck said, "You said," in a ten-year-old whine.

She said, "Don't you remember Cousin George?"

He frowned at me, screwing up one eye. Then he nodded. He was telegraphing: *Don't tell.* It was a game run according to playground conventions, with real guns. "Sure," he said. "I remember. I showed you my stamps."

"Great," I said.

"They didn't get my stamps," said Chuck. The Mannlicher was pointing at the ground now. I was sweating. There was music in the barn; Rhyd again, "Hole in a Lake."

I said, "I came to see the boys."

She said, "They're not here."

I stared at her. "So where are they?" I said.

"In camp," she said. "Camp, you know?"

"Where?" I said.

"Upstate. Pleasant Lake. They were messing around here, getting bored." She dropped her eyes. "And Chuck . . . well, he had a little turn. So I sent them up there."

I said, "You should have called."

She looked blank. "Why would I do that?"

There was no reason. The will had done the damage. She was a co-guardian, with the same rights as me. More: possession was nine points of the law. I said, "I'll go and see them."

She smiled. It was a tight little smile. She said, "That might not be real easy. They don't allow visitors in the settling-in period."

I thought of the grave hummocks in the lawn in front of the chapel. *Only the Brethren may penetrate the Tabernacle.* "It's a Brethren camp," I said.

"I am their guardian," she said. "It is my duty to see to their welfare. It's a real nice place."

I nodded, thinking of Chuck, and his guns, and his turns.

So was Sarah. Her eyes warmed a fraction. "I'm real sorry

about Chuck," she said. "Maybe it would be good if you were to call before you come down here. We had . . . an intrusion?"

"An intrusion?"

"Someone phoned," she said. "They told me there was a calf broke its leg up to Bullough Mountain. So Chuck and me went up there in the pickup. We didn't find any calf, but when we came back here, the front door was stove in and they'd been through the house."

"You mean you had burglars?" I said.

Chuck said again, "They didn't get my stamps."

"You can call them what you like," said Sarah. Her voice was becoming tighter, with a raw edge. "They went through the house, turned everything out of the closets, cast it around on the floors like junk." Her hands were shaking.

I said, "Did they take anything?"

"Couple of needleworks," she said. "Sacred texts. The police come. They said nothing's sacred any more." Her rawboned hands had been making little stabbing movements beside the hips of her drab print shirtwaister. She looked down at them, folded them in front of her.

"So they didn't catch them?"

"They were seen. There was a black man and a white man."

A black man and a white man had jimmied the Mustang's boot in Cambridge. Of course, there are a lot of black men and white men in America.

"Lieutenant Coleman reckoned there's been a couple of break-ins. They reckon we were lucky. Any road, I told Chuck he should be vigilant from now on. Maybe I overencouraged him a little."

"The boys weren't here," I said.

"They were here," said Sarah. "They came up with us to see the calf." She looked away. I guessed that the boys would have been making Chuck edgy and that the burglars would have been the final straw. "Elder Hornbeck gave them a ride to camp the day after. Now if you will forgive us, cousin, we have to regain our composure in the Lord."

"Of course," I said. Chuck was leaning against the trunk of the great maple in the yard. He had the grace of a bag of cement. "Can you give me the address of the camp?"

Sarah looked as if she was going to refuse. Then she said, "Sure," went into the house, and came out with a piece of paper. I tucked it in my pocket, turned the car around. When I looked in the rearview mirror, I saw Chuck standing thick legs astride in the driveway, ears sticking out under his cap, playing security guard. I waved to him. He waved back, halfheartedly, as if he had already forgotten me. Keeping the peace for his mommy and all the dead generations of Walterses since the *Ark*.

At the first corner I stopped and looked at the piece of paper. It said Pleasant Lake Camp. There was a Bangor post office box number. There was no other address. I stopped at the first public telephone. My hand shook as I dialed U.S. Mail in Bangor. They were sorry, sir, but it was contrary to regulations to divulge addresses behind box numbers, if any. A heavy weight of disappointment settled on me.

I looked in the index of the map. There were four Pleasant Lakes within fifty miles of Bangor. The schedule said I had another lecture tomorrow. This was no time for combing the rocks and trees of Maine for nephews who might have failed to answer my letters only because they had not received them. It was time I had a serious try at finding out what the hell Bill had been up to.

I stopped at a souvenir shop, bought a couple of postcards and sent them off. Then I headed south.

At six I drove into Quogue, parked, and walked down to the quay. As I passed Rooney's, the door opened. Danny's face was pinkish, as if someone had dripped grenadine into the cream. He said, "I saw ya on television."

I grinned back, and wondered what the polite formula was.

"Boy!" he said. "Them bastards did that to Rhyd, eh?"

"Bastards," I said.

"Telephone," he said, brandishing a slip of paper. "You wanna call from the restaurant?"

The number looked vaguely familiar. I dialed. A voice said, "Hello." Ricky Lee's voice. When she heard me, she said, "I found Sullivan."

"Great."

"Not great," she said. "He won't talk."

I said, "What do you mean?"

"He says Bill was a wild man, and Rhyd was crazy, and he has no idea about any story, and would I stop bugging him because he is an associate editor of *Woods and River* these days, and he thanks Christ he can hardly remember working for Serge Poliakoff." She coughed. "Serge has that effect on people."

I said, "Oh. Anything else?"

"Not on your story. I've been doing some interviews for the *Echo*. Real work. It's going great."

"Good," I said.

"But you don't care about that," she said. "I'm sorry. It's back to square one, huh?"

I found I did care about that. But I said, "That's right. What's the number?"

She gave me a number. She said, "He's a tricky guy. Tell me if you find anything out?"

I said, "I'll telephone."

I rang off. I dialed the Sullivan number. There was no reply, so I loaded myself into the dory and rowed out to the boat.

I thought about dead ends. I drank a beer, and thought more about dead ends. My ear was sore where Chuck had clocked it with his rifle.

I took out the paints. I made a quick picture of a pintail standing up in the water, beating its wings. It was not up to standard, but it had the customary soothing effect. At nine o'clock I turned out the lamp and rolled into the bunk, and fell asleep like a brick falling off a roof.

Sometime later, I found I was awake. I was awake in a peculiar way. My eyes had snapped open like mousetraps. I lay in the inky dark, listening to my heart beating like a bass drum under the distant nagging of whippoorwills.

And something else.

The tide was running past the hull with a steady gurgle. Wavelets were clocking against the side of the boat. They were falling out of rhythm with themselves, port side out of phase with starboard side. Up on deck, something creaked.

There was someone on board.

14

*I*T WILL BE SCOTCH JOHN, I THOUGHT. COME TO CHECK THINGS out.

It made sense, the way things make sense when you think you are awake but part of you is still asleep. Fingers fumbled at the hatch. It slid back, leaving a gray square of sky against which the fumbler was silhouetted. My heart stopped beating.

Scotch John was the shape of a concrete pillar, with a heavy mane of hair and a prophet's beard. The man silhouetted against the light had wide, chunky shoulders and a long jaw under a head that gleamed faintly, as if it had been shaved.

My heart cut in again with a thump. The man landed on the cabin sole quiet as a cat jumping off a chair. He had something in his hand. Gun, I thought. My mouth felt as if it was made of biscuit-fired clay. This is America. It could be a gun.

If you go up the steps, he will see you against the light, I thought. If you stay put, he will see you anyway.

The man lifted his right hand, the hand with the object in it. That's it, I thought, across the walloping in my chest. He's seen me.

A red light glowed on the object. There was an odd electronic crackling. The left arm reached for the bulkhead, in the general direction of the guitar locker.

I swallowed nothing. It was not a gun.

A locker door creaked open. The guitar-locker door.

I said, "This is a gun. Stand still."

He shouted. It must have been quite a shock. The red light went out. Something clattered on the deck.

A small-sized sun rose roughly where he was. Flashlight. I heard the scuffle of him moving away. I jumped out of the sleeping bag and dived at the flashlight.

Something very big and very hard hit me on the side of the head. My head rang like a church bell. Someone had taken the stuffing out of my knees. I went down sideways on to the cabin sole with an echoing crash. The flashlight beam swept around the cabin, glinted in the mirror. In it there appeared for a second a face: white, thickened at the nose and the lips, the cheekbones small and sharp and high above long, slablike cheeks. The face went. The feet sounded on the steps. The ringing in my ears had died to a buzz.

I went after him.

I came on to the deck swaying like a drunk. I could see him going over the lifelines. Must have a boat down there, I thought. Bastard. Clumsily, I fumbled for the boathook. I grasped it like an assegai and threw it at him. It hit him somewhere in the dark bulk of his body. He grunted, loud in the quiet night. A hard object clattered on deck. There was a small, definite splash. He turned around. Something about him moved, too quickly for me to be able to see what. I smelled garlic on his breath. Then something thumped me in the solar plexus and the night and the birds and the masts turned 360 degrees. My limbs belonged to someone else, and if I could have found anyone who wanted a pair of nonworking lungs, I would have given them mine.

The top lifeline was digging into my legs. I was leaning outboard, doubled up to protect my stomach. I leaned so far outboard that the wire tripped me. The night turned over. I went into the water in a sort of spraddled dive.

The water would have been cold enough to take my breath away, if I had had any breath to start with. I struggled, splashing. My face came above water. The lungs took an involuntary gasp of air. Better.

I reached for the side of the boat. My fingers found only water. I blinked the salt out of my eyes. I floated. What I saw left me paralyzed.

There was a half-moon above the gray water. There was a small rowing boat, black against a silver veil of fog, oars dipping untidily. Twenty yards away, there was the black silhouette of a moored ketch. I could not work out what had happened to *Halcyon*. The ketch seemed to be shrinking, foreshortening.

Then I realized.

The ketch was *Halcyon*. The ebb was running hard. If I kept floating like a dead pig, I was going to be washed out of the harbor. The fear was like another bang in the stomach. I tried to swim back toward the ketch. But my arms and legs felt weak. And I had started thinking. The sides were four feet high. There was no boarding ladder. The only way aboard was up the mooring pennant, and I was in no state for climbing mooring pennants.

To my left, a large, complex shape blackened the sky. For a moment, I had forgotten what it was. Then it came to me. It was Scotch John's houseboat.

The cold was intense. My fingers were losing sensation. One chance, Devis, I thought. I began to claw my way through the water, across the tide. My teeth were chattering in my head. All right, I thought. All right. The water was heavy as mercury. Keep going, I thought. If you go, it is all a dead end; in the village, for the boys. All in vain. I kept going.

My hand hit something hard. I emitted a whimper that was meant to be a curse. A black line crossed my horizon. The edge of something. The edge of a raft. The edge of the raft that housed Scotch John's collection of mongrel ducks. I heaved myself up on to the mat of evil-smelling straw.

There was a storm of quacking, and a rush of wings. I lay there with my face in something slimy.

A fuzzy voice said, "Who's that?"

I tried to answer. No sound came.

A door slammed. I passed out.

Sometime later, I must have tried to move my head. The muscles of my neck felt like rusty hawsers. My face was squashed into straw. I rolled over. My eyes creaked open. Under the belly of a duck, I saw a steaming metal plate and a red-hot ball of iron floating into darkness. It looked like dawn. Dawn. I crawled across the raft and on to the deck. A window opened. Scotch John's head looked out. "Jesus," he said. My mouth was a cave of dry mud. John helped me in. I drank half a gallon of water. He rowed me back to *Halcyon*.

When I awoke next, the cabin was hot and I was greasy with sweat. There was someone on deck again. I started shouting. Not much came out. A figure darkened the companionway hatch. This time, there was no mistaking the hair and the beard.

Scotch John said, "You just lie down."

I lay down. He clattered about with a kettle. I heard the rattle of what might have been the first-aid box. I swallowed pills, and a cup of coffee with something in it that burned. The aches in my ribs faded. I said, "You drugging me?"

"Heavy stuff," said John. "Paracetamol. Bourbon. You're all strung out."

I tried to grin at him. It hurt my neck.

He said, "So why were you hassling my ducks?"

My recollections were hazy. I said, "Burglars."

He said, "What did they take?"

I started to remember. I said, "Open the guitar locker."

He said, "It's open."

I craned my neck. It was painful, but it was working again. The locker door was ajar. It was empty. The urn had gone.

John said, "What's all this shit on the deck?" He was looking at his feet. The maple boards were filmed with a white dust. There was a little pile of the stuff in the corner. I remembered the curse, the clatter of something falling out of the locker.

Of the urn falling out of the locker.

The buzzing in my head was subsiding. The wheels of my mind meshed and began to clank. "Dustpan," I said. "Brush."

John went down on his knees and swept. I said, "Don't throw it away." I staggered on to my legs. My hands made crashing noises among the jars in the food locker and found an empty marmalade pot. "In here," I said.

He poured the contents of the dustpan into the jam jar. There was a good handful. I sat on the berth and waited for the blood to stop trying to hammer its way through the top of my skull.

John said, "What did he get?"

I did not answer. Last night was a movie with chunks hacked out of it. There was blackness. But at the end of blackness was an object clattering on deck. And something else.

John turned on the tap to rinse his hands. The water hit the aluminum sink with a heavy, thumping splash.

A splash.

I said, "Do you know any divers?"

"I can dive. I got gear." He made more coffee, no bourbon this time. He said, "So you went after this guy. And you fell overboard."

"That's right."

John shook his head. He said, "This is America. People can carry guns, even in the state of Maine."

"What would you have done?"

"Stayed quiet," he said. "You're lucky you ain't dead." He scratched his head. He said, "Someone bust into your car. And someone's bust into the boat. Everywhere you go, someone busts in. Right?"

My eyes felt like red-hot bullets. Someone had bust in at Bethel Bay, too.

"So they was looking for something. So whatever they took last night is what they was looking for. And now they got it, they will either leave you alone. Or."

Even with a headful of bilgewater, I knew what he was going to say, and I knew he was right.

"Or they know you know what they were looking for, and they will assume you are getting curious about why they wanted it. You have to assume the worst." He paused. "So what do you want dove for?"

"He dropped something overboard," I said. "Electronic device. Size of a Walkman."

He said, "I'll go fetch my gear."

He was back in a quarter of an hour wearing a wetsuit with a Day-Glo orange dive-leader's hood. I showed him where it might have fallen. He muttered about arcs of swing, shrugged into his tanks, and rolled backward into the gray-blue water.

Silver bubbles rose and burst. A couple of Arctic terns screamed. I waited.

I waited five and a half minutes by my Japanese Swiss watch. The cool wind worked magic on the hammers in my skull. As the second hand came around to thirty, the water erupted, and John's wet orange head cruised toward the boat. His right hand was raised. In the hand was a small black box, the size of a Sony Walkman. I took it. He shrugged his tanks into his inflatable, climbed on deck. "That it?" he said.

I looked at the little black box in my hand. Water was dripping out of a grill in its face, below a blank gray window that would have borne the numbers of an LCD. It said ZENITH 5–6000X. When I turned the on switch, nothing happened. Seawater and machines.

"Sitting by a rock," said John. "Thirty feet down. We were real lucky. Bottom's mud, smooth as a pool table. What is this?"

My headache was gone. My mouth was dry, and my hands were sweating.

CLAWHAMMER

Last night, this thing in my hand had made an electric crackling noise that had intensified with proximity to the urn.

I took his question in the general sense, not the particular. I said, "I don't know."

But in the particular sense, I did know.

The thing in my hand was a Geiger counter.

15

I SAID TO SCOTCH JOHN, "WHAT DO YOU KNOW ABOUT ETHIOPIAN flour?"

He combed his prophet's beard with his fingers. "Flour, zip," he said. "Dope, sure. Old Ethiopian saying: You want dope, try the cops or the Peace Corps; you want flour, try the UN."

So I pocketed the jam jar of flour and the soggy Geiger counter, climbed into the dinghy, and rowed very gently ashore. At the pay phone on the pier I called PKC. When I gave the operator my name, she put me through with gratifying speed. Pierce said, "How's it going?"

I told him it was going fine, ignoring the throb in my head.

"Lunch tomorrow?" he said.

According to the schedule, tomorrow was another senator's wife. I said, "Do you know anyone in the aid business?"

"Aid business?"

"Bags of corn to Third World countries."

"Oh." Pierce's voice lost its good-time-guy fizz and became the output facility of a machine built for making connections. "We met quite a few when we were on the Africa project. I'll see if Serge is free." He put me on hold for three minutes. "Try this," he said. "Charis Brown. She's on sabbatical from the FAO. Food and Agriculture Organization. Lives real close to where you are. Bar Harbor. She's a great lady. You'll like her. Serge says she's the best there is." He gave me the number. "It's a holiday cottage, but she's up there all year. Boat still afloat?"

"Still afloat."

He said goodbye. His voice was wandering. He was having a busy day, like all the other days in his life. We disconnected.

I called the number he had given me. A woman's voice said, "Who is this?" She sounded as if she was gargling gravel.

I told her who I was.

She said, "What do you want? How did you get my number?"

"Pierce Rapaport," I said.

"Oh, *Pierce,*" she said. Now she sounded like a dove gargling gravel. "So what can I do?"

I said, "I'd like to visit you for half an hour."

She told me where. I drank three large Cokes and ate four Tylenol. The head subsided. I climbed into the car and drove thirty miles northeast, then south again, across the green sound to Mount Desert Island. I passed among the august Edwardian villas of Bar Harbor. By mid-afternoon I was hammering on the door of a cedar-shingled bungalow with a view of what the map told me was Cadillac Mountain and a slice of Frenchman Bay. A dog was barking hysterically inside. Nobody seemed to have followed me.

The woman who opened the door was about sixty, wearing jeans, a checked shirt and a pink apron. Her hair was iron gray, cut in a short bob. Her eyes gleamed like chisels above heavy pouches. A spaniel wagged its tail ferociously at her feet.

"Ms. Brown?" I said.

"Miss Brown," she said. "You're the guy Rapaport sent? I guess you'd better come in."

There were floor-to-ceiling bookcases in the hall. There were more in the living room. There was a dusty wood stove and a grubby Navajo rug on the stained boards. It looked like the holiday cottage of a person who paid more attention to what she read than where she lived. She took off her apron, threw it in a corner and told me to sit down. I found a brown cord armchair facing a shelf of what looked like first editions of Konrad Lorenz.

"Well?" she said. She was standing in front of her fire, hands in pockets, moccasins planted apart on the rug.

The dog was a thin springer spaniel. It came and sniffed my foot. I patted it on the head, hoping to soften her. It did not work perceptibly. I said, "Food-aid corn. I need an expert."

She said, "I'm one." She frowned at me. "What did you say your name was?"

"George Devis."

"The ornithologist?"

"That's right."

Her heavy face lightened several notches. She took her hands out of her pockets. "I knew I'd seen you," she said. "On TV. Glad to meet you, George. Only Pierce sends the weirdest people sometimes. Journalists and like that. I very much admire your work on auks." She reached up, pulled down a volume from the top shelf. It was my *Auks* book. The *Best Guide to British Birds* was up there too. "So you can sign it for me."

I signed it.

She was fine, because she liked the books. And I was fine because someone had recognized me as something other than someone who had been on television. It was like being real again. She made tea, because she thought English people liked tea. We engaged in auk talk.

She said, "How did you meet Pierce? He's not an ornithologist."

I told her about the PloughShare campaign. She said, "That sounds more like it. Remarkable man, Serge Poliakoff. And Pierce even more so, in his way."

"In what way?"

146

"Summa cum laude, political science, Harvard. Wouldn't go into politics proper. Wrote his thesis on power, food and politics in the Baltic States, when there was a cold war. That was when I met him. Then he went and edited newspapers. And now he's working for this Poliakoff." Her mouth turned down at the corners.

I said, "You don't approve?"

She smiled. It was a tough, ironic, heart-of-gold smile. "No," she said. "In a way, I don't. Serge Poliakoff's a genius. But so were P. T. Barnum and Joe Stalin. He can afford to buy first-class minds. I don't like to see first-class minds being bought." She shrugged. "But then Pierce tells me I'm a silly old New England Democrat. I guess he could be right." She scratched a denim thigh. "I could go on all day, but I guess I'd better not. So you're interested in corn?"

"Food-aid corn," I said. "Pierce said you're an authority."

"Waste of time," she said.

"What is?"

"Food aid. Sending corn. There are big economic arguments against it, but I don't care about them. What I care about is the people end of it. They get dependent. Also, these places, you get tons of stuff coming off ships in an area miles away from the famine problem. All ports are corrupt. All Third World ports are entirely corrupt. So maybe three-quarters of the corn finds its way into the private markets. And the quarter that reaches its proper destination reinforces dependency on outside food sources."

I said, "Cynical."

She said, "Realistic." There was a silence. "All right," she said. "It's cynical. Out there you're dealing with cynical people in a cynical system. If you're not cynical, you get nowhere." She smiled again. Her teeth were strong and yellow. "So there you are," she said.

I said, "I want to ask you something in confidence."

She said, "People do it all the time."

She was strong-minded and matter-of-fact. I thought: You

can trust this woman. I said, "If a sample of corn sent to Ethiopia turned out to be radioactive, what would you think?"

She shrugged. "CIS probably," she said. "Russian, Ukrainian. They like to look good, and get rid of stuff they won't eat themselves. There's a lot of the Ukraine that glows in the dark."

"So you wouldn't be surprised?"

"Once you've been in the aid business, you don't surprise easy."

"How can I confirm it's Russian or Ukrainian or whatever?"

She picked a fat black filofax from beside the telephone, scribbled a number on a piece of paper. "Caroline Impey," she said. "Research grain scientist at the Wallace Institute in Portland. Tell her I sent you. I presume you've got a sample? Then come back to me, and we'll take it from there." She paused, head on one side. "Oh, by the way. Are you by any chance a White Knight?"

"A what?"

"White Knight. Solver of the world's problems. Like Poliakoff."

"No."

"They made you sound like one on TV."

I was feeling defensive. I said, "You can't get much done without publicity."

She made a surprising little-girl face, as if she had tasted something bitter. "There are no good causes," she said, handing me the piece of paper. "There are publicity stunts, and foul-ups. And experts. Caroline Impey's an expert."

"Can she keep her mouth shut?"

She said, "I guess. Excuse me for asking, but if you're not a White Knight, are you some kind of spook?"

"No," I said.

"Not that you'd tell me if you were," she said. "Well, I hope you're not. Magnet for spooks, the aid game." She shoved her hands into the pockets of her jeans, hunched her shoulders up into her grizzled bob. "Nice to meet you," she said. It was a dismissal, firm but fair.

I shook her by her hard, square hand, and set off into the afternoon. I liked Charis Brown.

The weather was closing in again, the blue of the sky dirty at the edges with fog creeping in from the sea. I stopped at a pay phone, dialed the number she had given me. When I dropped her name a secretary became very obliging. I arranged an appointment and climbed back into the car. The humidity was making it smell like a cardboard box in which someone had been living. At Ellsworth, I turned the nose on to Highway 1 toward Portland. Nobody seemed to be following. I shoved old coffee cups and hamburger cartons and sandwich wrappings into a carrier bag, in case I ran into a hitchhiker I wished to impress with the orderliness of my personality.

But there were no hitchhikers, only gray fog, and the ache of bruises. And a nasty, insecure feeling.

Bill Marsden had tried to smuggle radioactive flour across the Atlantic not to dodge Customs, but because he knew someone was after that flour. Bill Marsden was dead. And people were still looking for the flour. I remembered what Camilla had said, after Esias the silversmith had spoken of fire in the hills. *There comes a time when you can't not get involved.*

And she was dead, and Rhyd, and I had run away. But it was not a matter of obliterating the shame any more. The burglar had brought a message. The message was that I was involved too, up to my neck.

The fear came back: I recognized it. This time, I was in a civilized country. I told it to go to hell. For the moment, the rearview mirror stayed empty.

The Wallace Institute was an off-white box among pine-dotted lawns in the northern suburbs of Portland. The receptionist called up a secretary, who sent me to the back, where the carpets stopped and the corridors were clothed in green vinyl.

Dr. Caroline Impey was waiting outside a shatterproof glass door. She was wearing a white coat. She had mousy hair tied back in a thin ponytail, a prim oval face and pink eyelids. Her handshake was damp and flimsy. "Miss Brown says you have a problem," she said, avoiding my eyes. She led me into a laboratory. She said, "She gave you quite a buildup. How can we be of assistance?"

I shoved my hand into my coat pocket, brought out the jam jar of flour. I said, "I'd be interested to know where this comes from."

She took the jar in her hand, shook out a little flour. "Health food," she said. Her voice had become firmer, more confident. "Nope. Hold it." She tipped a pinch on to a microscope slide. "Interesting," she said. "It's loaded with rocks. Look." She beckoned me over to the binocular eyepieces.

The objective was filled with what looked like smashed-up fragments of wood. There were lumps of brown bark and chunks of dead-white heartwood, piled higgledy-piggledy on the slide. "Husk, germ and starchy portion," said Impey. "That's wholegrain flour. But look at those other guys." The other guys looked like big, dun-colored boulders. One of them had facets, like a crystal.

"Rocks," said Impey. "Stone-ground. But not with a big stone, the way it comes from a commercial mill. Look at the crushing on the grains. And the chunks of rock. Someone's pounded this in a hand mill. A quern, they call it your side of the Atlantic. Kind of pestle and mortar."

"Sure," I said.

"So it's from the Third World," she said. "Could that be right?"

I remembered the tall women with the faces of Egyptian queens and the babies bound on to their backs, laughing on the beaten earth in front of the mud houses, the ironwood pestles rising and falling. I remembered the dun-colored hills, the same dun as the miniature boulders in the microscope's objective.

I said, "Was it grown in the Third World, too?"

"Soon see," she said. Her voice had lost all trace of shyness. The hunt was up. "Let's try a little electrophoresis here." She took a pinch of flour and shook it up with distilled water in a test tube. Then she started making cabalistic movements with Bunsen burners and pipettes and an object that might have been an oscilloscope, except that it had a full-color screen and a little trapdoor on the top into which she dripped the flour-and-water mixture.

I said, "There's one other thing. It's radioactive."

"Radioactive?" She blinked at me with her pink lids. "That's bizarre. Russian, then, you think?" She pressed some buttons on the front of the machine. A blue line appeared on the screen. "There you are," she said, with the smugness of a conjuror from whose hat the rabbit has appeared without a hitch. "Electrophoretic signature. Hello." She frowned. "You said Russian."

"Yes," I said.

"Uh-uh," she said, shaking her head. She was looking through me, consulting her inner catalogs. "You're looking at a North American hard wheat here. Grown in the Midwest, maybe Canada."

"So what was it doing in Ethiopia?"

"Someone shipped it there," said Impey. "Aid or trade. There's no way of telling."

No way of telling. American wheat, hand-milled and reimported from Ethiopia in the urn intended for my brother-in-law's ashes. People were committing crimes to get hold of it. I said, "How did it get radioactive?"

She shrugged. She said, "Accidentally. On purpose. Who knows? It's not my field."

We chatted for a couple of minutes about the weather. Her shyness had returned. I got the feeling she wanted to get rid of me. As far as she was concerned, the problem was solved.

Finally, I said, "Do you know anyone who . . . knows about radioactivity?"

She frowned. "I could make inquiries, if you liked. Why?"

"I'm curious," I said.

She said, "I'll do my best."

I said, "Thank you."

We divided the contents of the jar into two plastic bags. I kept half. She gave me a receipt for the other half in her neat, precise handwriting.

I left Portland, heading south. I watched the rearview mirror all the way.

16

I FOUND A MOTEL IN A LOOP OF ROAD NORTH OF HIGHWAY 95 halfway between Portland and Boston. The Mustang stood out from the Toyotas like an orange in a pile of coal. I parked it around the back of the cabins, paid cash at the office, and headed for the telephone.

Ricky Lee answered on the third ring. I found I was pleased to hear her voice, and she sounded pleased to hear mine. She said, "I just interviewed Randy Newman. Now I have a gig at the Colonial Inn. I feel ridiculous."

I said, "Break a leg."

She said, "Why, thank you," in a deep Southern accent. It was good to hear someone make a joke, even a little one.

I said, "Do you have Sullivan's address?"

She said, "Sure. He's not there."

"Or he's not answering the phone."

"Maybe." She sounded vague, as if her mind was on the forthcoming ordeal at the Colonial.

"Could you give it to me?"

"Why?" Her voice had cooled. It reminded me that she was a

journalist as well as a folksinger. Journalists do not get to the top by sharing their contacts.

"I want to write to him."

"Okay." She left me hanging on. "260 Ellerton. In Cambridge, off Mass. Avenue, north of Harvard Square."

I thanked her, hung up. Then I lay and stared at the acoustic tiles on the ceiling.

Radioactive American wheat, shipped to Ethiopia, brought back by Bill. It sounded like evidence.

I rolled out of bed at three A.M., showered, and pointed the Mustang south. It was still dark, but the sky was lightening as I turned off 94 and dived into Cambridge.

Cambridge is the northern half of Boston. Ellerton Street was quiet and leafy and empty. The houses were built of brick that might have been brown; it was hard to tell in the half-light. Birds in the maples were raising the raucous din that passes for a dawn chorus in America. I drove past number 260 slowly. The little front yard was unkempt, the blinds drawn. That was a good sign. People who go away do not draw their blinds. Drawn blinds attract burglars.

I parked the Mustang and walked back to the house. The lemon-colored glow in the eastern sky reflected in the glass of the front window. I put my thumb on the bell.

I heard it ring. There was no movement. I rang again.

A dog began to bark: a sharp yowf, a big terrier or a small gundog. Gotcha, I thought. People who go away may forget to draw their blinds, but they do not forget to take their dog.

There were feet on the stairs, a snuffling. A voice inside the door said, "What do you want?"

I said, "Police."

A man's voice grunted. It sounded half-asleep. A chain rattled. The door opened.

I walked into the hallway. I had not expected to get this far. I stayed mute. Not many Boston policemen have English accents.

He said, "What time is it?" He was squinting at me. I was

wearing an assortment of navy blue clothes. I needed a haircut. I did not look like a mugger.

I said, "Early." There was no light in the hall. I tripped over something. In the half-darkness it looked like a pair of suitcases and a tube of the kind people use for carrying fishing rods.

Sullivan was a big man bulging halfway out of the bath towel around his waist. His arms and legs were covered in reddish hair. There was red hair on his head over a drinker's face, creased with sleep, suspicious and bleary at the same time. He smelled as if he might not have gone to bed sober. If he had, he would not have let me in at the door. He said, "Let's see your ID."

I pulled out my wallet, opened it, snapped it shut. He did not look as if he was seeing too well. He said, "Hold it. I'll get a bathrobe."

I heard him moving about upstairs. There was the murmur of a voice. When he came down the voice continued: a radio. He grunted, led the way into a kitchen and switched on a harsh fluorescent light. There were two empty Gallo Burgundy bottles, one dirty plate. He switched on a kettle with a blow of his fist. He said, "So what do you want?"

I said, "You were working with Bill Marsden." The accent was terrible.

He shoveled instant coffee into a mug, tipped in water that had not boiled. He did not offer me any. "So?"

I said, "Bill's dead."

He brought the coffee cup down from his face. "I know," he said. His eyes were gummy, but suspicious. "You're not a cop," he said.

I said, "I'm a friend of Bill's. You were an editor of the *Echo*."

He said, "What the fuck—"

I said, "Bill's dead. You're off fishing. Unless I call the cops. Then you'll be a material witness, and they will want you to be answering questions."

He stared at me with his mouth open. He shut it. He said, "You and Ricky Lee Klaasen."

"That's right."

"You a goddamn folksinger, too?"

"No."

He sat down at the table and scratched his coarse hair. "Marsden and Klaasen," he said. "Clever as hell. But no goddamn respect."

I said, "What exactly was Bill Marsden doing for you?"

"Filing expenses claims," he said. "Tickets all over Africa, Europe. The *Echo*'s a Boston paper, for chrissakes. Long Island's overseas. And there's Marsden in frigging Ethiopia."

I said, "What was he doing there?"

He held up a wine bottle, grimaced at its emptiness, gulped his coffee mixture instead. He laughed. "You think Marsden'd tell a simple editor what story he was working on?" He screwed up one eye. " ' 'Lo, Sullivan. Can't talk right now. Aid crime. Ethiopian politics. Hillbilly music tapes. Sign the expenses sheet.' "

Everything had gone quiet. The dawn chorus continued, but against a new kind of silence. I said, "Hillbilly music?"

"Someone sent me a tape," he said. "From England. Bill said, when you get the tape, guard it with your life. Some hillbilly singer. Personally I am into Wagner, and he knew it."

I said, "Have you still got it?"

He said, "Sure."

I said, "Could I hear it?"

He looked at the stainless-steel Rolex on his hairy wrist. He said, "At seven o'clock I am going to Logan and getting on a plane, and the plane is taking me away from goddamn Boston trout fishing in Kashmir, on assignment for *Woods and River*, on which I have been invited to become a contributing editor after thirty years hacking it out for one goddamn scandal sheet after another. This is the culmination of my ambitions, because it means I am being paid for going fishing. If you think I am hanging around listening to hillbilly music, you are out of your fucking mind."

I said, "That cassette is material evidence in a murder case.

Like I said, you could be talking to the police. But you'd miss your plane."

He looked at me from his bleary eyes. He looked at me for a long time, as if he were adding things up. He walked over to a desk. I heard him clattering through junk. "Here," he said. "You like it, you have it."

He handed me a padded envelope addressed to him in Bill's handwriting. There was a cassette case in the envelope. There was a cassette in the case. "Part two," he said.

"Part two?"

"He was bringing over something," said Sullivan. "Part one. Together with this tape, part two. It was evidence for something, parts one and two. Do not ask me what, because I neither know nor care."

I said, "Thank you."

He said, "You're welcome."

I slid the tape into my pocket. I said, "Tight lines," and let myself out of the door.

The sun was up. The leaves on the maples looked young and fresh. The sky was clear blue and the street was empty, except for a bum shuffling down the sidewalk toward me. The bum was wearing a dirty parka with a hood. Inside the parka, his shoulders looked as wide as a barn door. When he was thirty yards away, he glanced at me.

My heart rolled in my chest.

He had high cheekbones, a flat nose, lips mashed back over his teeth. I had seen the face before. It was the face reflected in the shaving mirror as the flashlight beam swept across *Halcyon*'s saloon. The face of the man who had taken the urn.

I pulled the cassette out of my pocket and dropped it into the hedge that separated Sullivan's yard from the road. He did not see me do it. I took the two steps back to the front door, leaned on the bell. The dog started yapping inside. A voice from upstairs shouted, "Screw *you!*"

I opened my mouth to shout.

A voice said, "No noise."

I turned around.

The man in the parka was standing at the bottom of the garden path. He was smiling. He said, "Spare change, boss?"

I said, "Go to hell."

His hand came out of his pocket. A blade was growing from a lumpy fist. He said, "Throw me your wallet."

I leaned on the bell again.

He came up the path in two strides. I aimed a punch at his face. He caught my wrist, yanked my arm up between my shoulder blades, dragged me down the path so we were behind the hedge. His parka was hanging open. He was wearing gray sweat pants and a T-shirt bearing the device of a big black fist in a boxing glove. His face was very close, so I could see the little silvery scars of old ring-cuts on his brow-ridge. He said, "Doan get clever wit me. Turn out your pockets." The knife was under my chin. I could feel the sharp point of it digging upward. One shove, I thought. Through the soft palate into the brain. And the boys are on their own, and everything I know is no use to anyone.

The fear was back.

I turned out my pockets: wallet, keys, loose change.

He backed away. He squatted down, kept his eyes on my face, spread the stuff out on the sidewalk, sorted it by touch. He leafed through the wallet, took $150 dollars. He picked up the car keys, threw them down the road into someone else's garden. I marked them, moving only my eyes.

He got up, walked toward me. When he was six inches away he said, "Turn around. Put up your hands."

My skin crawled. I could smell his breath mints. The point of the knife stung my belly. I turned. This is it, I thought. Goodbye. Nothing you can do.

He frisked me, a quick, professional job. There was nothing else to find. He was looking for the tape, I thought. Part two, the tape. Fitting part one, the urn. How did he know?

He finished the shakedown. He stood away. Now it comes, I thought.

Something slammed into my backbone. It felt like a train.

The breath whooshed out of me. My legs buckled, and I went down. I found myself deeply interested in whether my spinal column was cut and whether I would ever breathe again.

Miles away, someone said, "Keep out of it."

Red clouds misted my brain. I rolled. My knees were up by my chin. I waited for the pain. The pain came. After a very long time, it faded. With the fading, oxygen leaked back. My toes moved. Spinal column fine. I rolled on to my knees.

The mugger was gone.

I crawled to my wallet. I crawled over and pulled the tape out of the hedge. I crawled down the road to the garden where the keys had gone and hunted around. A jogger jogged by, eyes carefully averted. The keys were lying by the gatepost.

I crawled back to the bell and rang it. Nobody came. Thank you, Mr. Sullivan. I crawled into the car. I drove away, slumped against the door, breathing as little as possible.

When I could think at all, I thought about muggers.

I thought about a mugger who was also a burglar.

Very few people had known I was visiting Mr. Sullivan. Mr. Sullivan knew; and Mr. Sullivan had turned on his radio, possibly to mask the sound of the telephone call he had made.

The only other person who knew I knew where Sullivan lived was Ricky Lee Klaasen, who said she knew nothing about the story Bill Marsden had been working on. But Ricky Lee was an ambitious journalist. And I had only Ricky Lee's word for the fact that she knew nothing about the Bill Marsden story.

I decided not to visit Ricky Lee just yet.

I checked into a motel. I called Sullivan's number. There was no answer. It sounded as if he had made it to the airport. I lay on the bed for a couple of hours, unstiffened the back in the shower. Soon it did not hurt to breathe.

When I could raise my arms high enough, I climbed into the suit and the black shoes and slogged back the hundred-odd miles to Portland, where I was due to speak in the house of Mrs. Senator Harry Chance. On the way I played the tape, and kept my eye on the rearview mirror.

There was nothing in the mirror that should not have been there. There was nothing on the tape, either.

It was a standard Rhyd sent-home-from-Africa tape: guitar, bass, synthesizer, some mandolin; Rhyd singing a bunch of laconic country songs, Camilla on some high harmonies. I was not in top intellectual form, but it did not sound in any way out of the ordinary. And hearing Camilla's voice made me think about her, which made me sad. And feeling sad made me think about the fear . . .

I wrenched my mind back. Bill had not been a madman, whatever anyone said. The tape was part two, and the flour was part one. The tape was information.

I concentrated on the difficult art of painless breathing. Save your energy for the guests of Mrs. Senator Harry Chance, Devis. Try again later.

At the lunch, there were the usual cameras, the usual old women. I kept thinking about muggers.

I looked them over carefully, diamonds and hairdos and dewlaps. I told myself that none of these people was going to pull a machine gun and tear my head off. But tell myself as I would, I had to keep my hands in my pockets to hide their shaking.

I did the speech. I drank the refreshing glass of Chardonnay and did not make faces when the back hurt me. The donations were safely gathered in. The people went away. Pierce Rapaport came up to me. He was wearing a beautiful tweed jacket, corduroy trousers with a razor-sharp crease, and a nice quiet bowtie in autumnal reds and browns.

"Going great," he said.

I managed a grin.

He frowned, looked at my hand. I looked too. The hand was shaking. "Are you okay?"

I said, "Fine." Pierce exuded confidence and *savoir vivre*, in keeping with the drawing room of Mrs. Senator Harry Chance, in which we were sitting. There was a senatorial Matisse on the wall. Outside the French windows, a senatorial garden by

Lanning Roper unrolled a vista of yew hedges and a Florentine fountain into a pearly limbo of fog. I shifted my weight to ease the pain in my back.

Pierce said, "Did you hurt yourself?"

I told him I had been mugged. The words sounded as if they might cause the flower arrangements to wilt.

Pierce rested his brown eyes on me. He looked worried. He said, "I'm sorry to hear that."

I made a decision. I said, "Let's take a walk."

Pierce followed me through the French windows, down the yew alley and into a rose garden. His beautiful shoes were wet with dew. I said, "This was not a straightforward mugging."

He said, "What do you mean?"

I said, "Someone is after something I've got."

Pierce stopped by a rose bush next to a greenish pond. It was too early in the year for roses, but this one had spent its youth in a hothouse. "What is it that you have got?" he said.

"A sample of flour. A tape of songs."

"Ah," said Pierce.

"American flour," I said. "Bill was bringing it back from Ethiopia. It was part of the story he was working on."

Pierce picked a rose. It looked like a Dutch Portrait. Camilla had planted one by the barn, a thousand years ago, a million miles away. He said, "Listen, George. I'm going to suggest something a little out of line here. I know you are . . . interested in finding out the whys and wherefores of this situation."

I said, "That's right."

He said, "So am I. From a journalistic point of view." He sniffed the rose. "And others."

I said, "So put a team on it."

He said, "It's not quite as easy as that. Serge owns a lot of things. Not just newspapers and TV stations. I work for Serge. I give him total commitment. He pays me very well. He sees his corporations as a totality, different segments of a machine for making money. And of course, so do I." He paused. His face had an expression I had not seen before. He looked worried, racked with self-doubt. "Up to a point. Can I speak . . . confidentially?"

It was thanks to Pierce that I had got this far. I said, "Of course."

He was pulling the rose apart now. The blood-red petals landed in the green water of the pond. The wind scooted them to the downwind side, where they piled up until the ripples sank them. "I am not paid for nothing. In this situation, we have arrived at a . . . commercial impasse. There are facts I think we should publish that can't be published, because of commercial pressures from elsewhere in the group. So I can't ask anyone in the group to go looking."

"Facts?"

He allowed his sharp eyes to rest on me. He said, "This will interest you. Someone you know flew into Seattle yesterday."

"Who?"

"Ras Hamil."

I stared at him. I said, "What's he doing here?"

"He's on an . . . inspection trip. Serge hopes to become his partner in certain . . . nonjournalistic ventures."

I said, "What does that mean?"

Pierce's face was still. "It means he invited him here," he said. "I think that you might have had something to do with that."

I said, "Me?"

"You won a race."

I remembered Poliakoff after the race. *Wait and see.* I said, "That would have been quick."

Pierce said, "It is easy to underestimate the power Serge can bring to bear in . . . certain areas."

I said, "What are you talking about?"

Pierce grinned, a grin whose naturalness was surprising in his well-schooled face in the mannered garden. He said, "Serge believes that if this man is a contender to run Ethiopia, Serge can sell him products that he makes in his factories. If you run a country, even a country like Ethiopia, you have materials to trade. Trade is what Serge is about."

I said, "So why ask him over for my sake?"

"For Serge's sake," said Pierce. "That's the only sake he ever does anything for. He likes a competition. You against General Hamil. If Hamil's no good, you'll beat him. If he is any good, he'll beat you. Serge only deals with winners. See?"

I said, "Why would he be underwriting a lecture tour that is damaging Hamil?"

Pierce smiled, his courtier's smile. "You must remember that it is not Serge Poliakoff's way to be seen to curry favor with Third World despots."

In the clammy New England rose garden, a polite little jet of water was tinkling out of a stone dolphin's mouth. I could feel the Ethiopian sun pressing like a hot anvil on my head; smell the harsh, bitter smell of burned mud and thatch. The old man had stopped talking. The young man was there with his round, smiling face, the frizz of hair perched on the back of his skull like a yarmulke, his right eye squinting firmly inward at his nose. *It is Ras Hamil who has done this.* And I had called up Derek, and flown away, scared out of my wits.

I said, "What are you trying to say?"

He said, "It can be a problem, running a news outfit which is a subsidiary of a powerful industrial outfit. One has to . . . fight one's corner. Pick one's causes. Let's say that I think you and I can do good things together. I'm talking about me personally. Serge is using you as window dressing. I think we can go further, bring a little old-fashioned justice to bear on this man Hamil. What I am offering . . . personally, now and above my corporate duty . . . is a measure of informed support."

I thought about Charis Brown. I said, "You're already providing that. You'll get your story. But it doesn't sound as if you'll be allowed to publish it."

Pierce said, "I wasn't thinking of publishing it as a regular story."

"Then what?"

"As an investigation, leading to an indictment," said Pierce. "For the murder of Rhydian and Camilla Walters. Rhydian Walters was a U.S. citizen. His murderer can be tried under U.S. jurisdiction."

I stared at him.

He said, "Serge Poliakoff is a powerful man. But he's not as powerful as the Justice Department."

The silence expanded to fill the garden. There was a voice in my mind. Camilla's voice. *You can't not get involved.* And apart from that voice, nothing. The scratchy little voice of my conscience was stilled.

"Well?" he said. He was not smiling any more. His eyes were narrow. "It could be dangerous. We'll have to find you a bodyguard."

From out of the quiet, I heard my own voice say, "That will be fine."

17

*W*HEN I ARRIVED AT QUOGUE, IT WAS EIGHT O'CLOCK, AND THE sun was dropping toward the water. I parked the Mustang by the quay and took a slow, careful look around. There were gulls sitting on the mooring posts, an old man mumbling at a lobster trap he was mending, a forklift loading crates of farmed salmon into a refrigerated van.

I pulled my bag out of the car and walked down to Rooney's. Danny was hauling a plate of deep-fried clams to a family of early tourists in one of the booths. It was all fine, and safe, and normal.

I said, "Any letters?"

"Nope. Phone messages, is all."

"Oh." Camp or no camp, the boys should certainly have written by now. You were down there in Boston, I thought. You should have found a lawyer.

But there was an ache in my back and a nervous twitch in my eyes that explained exactly why I had not been looking for lawyers.

Danny handed me a slip of paper with two numbers on it

and waved me to the telephone. I dialed the first. The voice on the other end was gravelly and familiar. "Miss Brown," I said.

"Charis," she said. "Look, Caroline Impey wants to talk. She met with a radiologist, I think. She's all excited. She's so excited she won't talk on the phone. Can you get over here tomorrow? Early afternoon?"

"Fine," I said, and rang off. The second number was Ricky Lee's. I had been thinking about Ricky Lee, and how the man in the parka had found me on Ellerton Street at four A.M.

She said, *"Hi!"* Her voice was bright as champagne.

I said, "You rang."

"I had some news," she said. "At least, I wanted to thank you. They gave me a job."

"Who did?"

"The *Echo.* I'm a probationary staff reporter. Real ambulances to chase. Real money. I guess it was that PloughShare stuff. We should have a drink. Two drinks."

The warmth of her voice reminded me that there were such things as friends and going to bars with good-looking women who were interesting to talk to. That was how I had felt last time we had spoken. I had to remind myself sharply that in my present situation I needed to be quite certain whose side the good-looking women were on. I said, "Another time. I'm in Maine."

She said, "That's a pity." She sounded properly disappointed. "Did you write to Sullivan?"

I said, "I went to visit him."

She said, "He let you in?"

"I told him I was a cop."

"An English cop?" she laughed. "That guy can really drink. What did he give you?"

I looked at the picture of Rhyd with the lobster claw in his hat band. "Nothing," I said. "He didn't know what I was talking about."

"Oh," she said. "I'm sorry." The disappointment sounded authentic. I wanted to be convinced. "You take care," she said. "I worry."

I laughed. It hurt my back.

"So . . . call soon," she said.

She sounded as if she wanted to. But it could have been her who had told whoever it was had alerted the boxer in the parka.

Time would tell.

I climbed down the quay and paddled out to the boat. John had been over and tidied up. The last traces of flour had gone from the deck and the ropes were in neat ammonite coils. I sat there for a minute, looking out to sea. The scaup was taking her children for a swim. The same old sun was falling into what looked like the same old fogbank. Anyone who had had a different forty-eight hours from me would have been thinking deep and peaceful thoughts.

Personally, I was frightened.

A lot of things frighten me. Heights, for instance. Fear of heights is rational, because if you fall off something high, you land up dead. The sea does not frighten me, and nor do traffic accident statistics. If having taken precautions you drown or are hit by a truck, you are unlucky. Fear of bad luck is paranoia, not self-preservation.

What was frightening me now was a fear descended from the one I had felt in the village in Africa. It was the fear of being on the fringes of a great big machine that encompassed muggers in Cambridge and burglars on boats, and olive-drab trucks that machine-gunned and burned Rhyd and Camilla. It was working silently, the machine. I was not even sure it existed. But I had to find it, and crawl into its works, and take it apart. Starting tomorrow.

A dory was coming across the water. The rower was big enough to bulge over the sides. John.

He turned his head. He said, "Howdy."

I was reassured by the quiet voice across the flat sea.

He said, "You want to go for a beer?"

"No." I wanted to sit somewhere nice and quiet and think about the machine.

John pulled a length of cord out of his overall pocket. He had started something that was undoubtedly going to be one of his Turk's heads. His crowbar fingers moved at blinding speed. The one-dimensional string became two-dimensional, then three. "You get the end," he said. "And you work it out." He looked at me. His black eyes were clear and steady. "How are you doing?"

He was not asking about the state of my health. I said, "The guy who killed Rhyd. Poliakoff's flown him into the States. Maybe we can make out a case against him."

"Here?"

"Apparently."

He combed his grizzled beard with his fingers. "All *right,*" he said.

I said, "How are you on bodyguarding?"

He looked down at the knot. "I never tried."

"Could you start tomorrow?"

His teeth showed in his beard. "Sure," he said.

"And now you can maybe tell me where I can anchor up where nobody can find me."

He shoved the knot back into his pocket and pointed out a bay on the chart, tucked into an island with no roads. I slung the hook, motored around the corner into the gray dusk and anchored in the bay. There were no other boats, no lights ashore, ten thousand birds. I drank a beer. Ordinarily, I could happily have spent till full dark sorting out the ducks from the gulls from the waders. Not tonight. I was thinking about being in the same country as Ras Hamil.

I was tired, but I slept badly and woke at dawn. The ketch was floating in a silver void of fog. I started the engine and motored on a succession of compass bearings back to Quogue harbor.

John was fishing beside the Ping-Pong table in the tug's well. It was a quiet morning; metal, sea, fog in giant cushions outside the harbor. I picked up the mooring buoy.

He said, "We going?"

I said, "Yes, please."

He was three hundred yards away. Neither of us had raised our voices, but the sound crossed the water clear as a bell.

He said, "I'll just water the vegetables."

John fed the ducks on his raft, vanished below, reappeared, clambered into his dory and rowed over. "Climb aboard," he said.

I climbed aboard. "Nice, John," I said.

He looked vaguely sheepish, and started to row. He had on a sports coat that had been built for someone smaller than him in claret-and-Day-Glo-green acrylic plaid. His white nylon shirt failed by two inches to encompass his neck. He was wearing a black leather tie and a pair of Levis. He had greased his hair savagely. The effect was of a Viking on his way to play golf. It looked bizarre, but it also looked dangerous.

"Thanks for coming," I said.

"Cool," he said, relaxing visibly. I drove the forty miles to Bar Harbor, then out of town, into the woods and into the driveway of the shingled house of Charis Brown.

I said, "I won't be a minute."

John said, "Who's in there?"

"Lady college professors."

"Do they carry knives?"

"Not big ones."

He grinned. He pulled his piece of string from his pocket. His fingers began working. "Good luck," he said.

Charis Brown was still in checked shirt and jeans, but without an apron. She was in the room with the bookshelves. Caroline Impey was with her. Dr. Impey's hair was untied, curly and blond. Her mouth was prim, her eyes nervous under the pink lids. It was just as well John had stayed in the car. We shook hands. Charis's was warm and firm. She seemed genuinely pleased to see me. "Dr. Impey thought I should be here to . . . well, referee. And I may be able to cast some light." She smiled on Dr. Impey, who smiled back, a small, nervous smile, and dropped her eyes. "Now," she said, "Caroline. Can you tell us?"

Dr. Impey blinked, like a mouse that has arrived on a stage at the moment someone has turned on the spotlights. She said, "I can't think why anyone should have done it."

Charis Brown said, "Done what?"

"Irradiated this sample."

Charis Brown said, firmly but without exasperation, "Would you care to start at the beginning?"

I was beginning to see that she would have made a remarkably effective committee person. Dr. Impey fluttered her pink eyelids and seemed panic-stricken. I said, "So you've made progress?"

It was a handle. She pursed her lips, raised her mouselike chin, and said, "Certainly. I subjected portions of the sample to a range of tests and analyses—"

"I'm afraid we're not familiar with the terminology," I said. She began to look like a mouse with feelings of superiority. "Could you just give us an outline of your conclusions?"

She smiled faintly, raised her chin. She said, "In layman's terms, then. Radioactivity is the emission of ionizing radiations, detectable by a range of devices. In the case of a sample contaminated by accident, say, there would be many radioactive signatures, as we may call them." Charis Brown stifled a yawn. Her eyebrows were low over her heavily pouched eyes. She was not taking kindly to the undergraduate-lecture form of address. "But this sample is different. In this sample, there is only one element present. I assume it to be a radioactive isotope of iodine." She paused. It was a significant pause. Intelligent undergraduates were invited to prod her.

I filled it. I said, "So what can we deduce from this?"

She began to look like a mouse hot on the scent of cheese. She said, "Radioactive isotopes of iodine have a range of beneficial characteristics. Like all isotopes, they can serve as markers."

"Markers?"

"As in tracking mechanisms. Possibly as X-ray-visible markers for use in the human body; to show, for instance, lymphatic obstructions. Iodine is specifically useful in agriculture. Spray it on a growing plant and the produce of that plant will be nontoxically marked—*specifically* marked—until it is destroyed. I think we can hypothesize that your flour sample has been milled from corn thus marked." She sniffed, a mouse on her dignity. "Though as I said at the beginning of this seminar—conversation—I have absolutely no idea why."

I caught her eye, smiled at her. She smiled back, looking a little flustered. I said, "Thank you very much for this penetrating analysis, Doctor."

She said, "It has been a pleasure." For a moment, she looked as if it had.

Miss Brown said, "So someone put a trace on some corn. And we don't know who or why."

Dr. Impey said, "That's right."

I said, "Charis, do you have any ideas?"

She shrugged. She said, "I told you last time we met. Aid and spooks go together like beans and cornbread. I'm not interested in spooks."

Dr. Impey found herself suddenly on the margin of the conversation. She smiled helplessly, her eyes shuttling between us. I had the impression that there was something else she wanted to add, but that she was not sure if it was allowed. Finally, she said, "Excuse my asking, but are you by any chance the George Devis who wrote the *New Eclogues*?"

For a moment I was disappointed. Then I was nonplussed, the way a football-playing surgeon might be nonplussed if someone kicked a football at him while he was operating. "Yes," I said. "That's me."

She bit her prim bottom lip. The assurance of her home ground had left her. She said, "Would you . . . I mean, we have a poetry society at the college. We meet weekly, for readings. Tonight . . . well, I expect you're busy."

Under normal circumstances, poetry societies give me the creeps. These were not normal circumstances. I said, "I'd be delighted to come."

Her whole face turned pink as her eyelids. She said, "That would be *wonderful!* We meet in the Wyeth Room at the U. at six-thirty? There's a glass of wine available. Charis, why don't you come?"

Charis Brown said, "Portland's too far for poetry. Even George's."

"Oh, but you should *try,*" said Dr. Impey. "Now, I have to get back."

I said, "See you later, Doctor."

She said, "Caroline." She left.

Charis Brown shook my hand. Her grip was hard and uncompromising. She said, "That was an altruistic little gesture."

I said, "Equal parts vanity and curiosity."

"Of course." She did not let go of my hand. "George, I have formed a good opinion of you. I would not like to see you get hurt."

I said, "What do you mean?"

She said, "Someone has gone to a lot of trouble to mark this corn. An unusual amount of trouble. A wise person might let sleeping dogs lie."

"Aid and spooks?" I said.

"Precisely."

I grinned at her. "Thank you," I said.

Her eyes were worried. "But you won't stop asking questions?"

"Eventually," I said.

"Come visit?"

"Of course."

And I went outside, back on to the one-way street to the heart of the machine.

18

*I*N THE CAR, JOHN LOOKED UP FROM THE LANYARD VIA WHICH HE had been investigating the secrets of the universe. "Where to, boss?" he said.

"Portland," I said. "Let's get something to eat."

The gearshift felt different. John had covered the knob with an elaborate knot. We stopped at a greasy spoon. I ordered a steak and a salad; athlete's food in the face of ordeal by verse. John ordered bacon, eggs, sausages and the Stack O'Pancakes All Day Breakfast Special, and doused the works with synthetic maple syrup.

"Pure energy," he said. He ate in silence. Afterward he pulled his string from his pocket and we went back to the car.

I shoved Rhyd's tape into the machine again. The rocks and trees unreeled. Camilla used to play a nylon-string guitar and had cultivated a Joan Baez vibrato. When we had lived in the Sweigh house, I had written songs for her: poets' songs, too clever by half. Rhyd had not approved. But he had worked on Camilla's sense of rhythm. And now there they were, on the player, singing a song about an early aviator making a forced landing:

> Look out that window, Mavis,
> Did Gabriel blow his horn?
> It's worse than that there, Elmer,
> There's a birdman in the corn.

The birdman ran off with the farmer's daughter. The farmer had been angry about the crop the plane had destroyed, but he was sad about losing his daughter. It was not in the mainstream of Rhyd's songs.

It was just double-tracked guitar, bass, no banjo or fiddle. I thought I had heard it before somewhere, with a banjo track, clawhammer-style. I could not remember where. It did not matter where. What mattered was that this was part two. Whatever that meant.

We listened to it twice. There were three songs. There was "Birdman in the Corn," which was innocuous. There was a song called "Mr. Coffee," a sort of come-all-ye about an apocalyptic visitor to a village. That sounded more like it. But the words were nonspecific, devoid of facts. And finally, there was a version of "The Alleluia Tree."

It was the same old "Alleluia Tree." But on this version, there was a verse tacked on to the end.

> When the Book of Life is written
> To which this is the key,
> The Lord will post it in the library
> By the Alleluia Tree.

That sounded more like information. But the Alleluia Tree was in Ethiopia. And what the Book of Life was I did not know. Perhaps it would have meant something to Bill.

I popped out the tape and tried to remember how you have a poetry reading.

We arrived at the university at six and parked in a lot around the corner from the Wallace Institute. Caroline Impey met us at the door of the Wyeth Room. She was wearing a dark green pinafore dress with a pink polo neck. Her smile faded when she saw John's golf jacket and leather tie. "An associate," I said. "World authority on marine ropework."

John showed his teeth in his beard and Caroline Impey's eyes took in the Turk's head on his wrist. "Ah," she said. "Now, then. I could only find about fifty people, I'm afraid."

Fifty was an outrageously good crowd at two hours' notice. They sat in a horseshoe-shaped lecture theater. I read from the library copy of the *New Eclogues*. They stayed awake throughout and asked questions afterward.

"The pastoral motifs," said a man with thick glasses. "What proportion of these is based on direct personal observation?"

I tried to remember. But between me and the pastoral motifs heaved an Atlantic of blood.

At the end, Dr. Caroline Impey was delighted. Her stock had evidently rocketed. We went to the faculty bar. She had darkened her pink eyelids. She looked at me over her glass of Chardonnay like a mouse who had unexpectedly found the key to the porridge drawer.

"That was great," I said.

"For us also," she said. "Can you come again?"

"Say the word."

"We will." She smiled. "I have to get back to my husband. He doesn't like poetry. He doesn't know what he's missing." She blushed, became businesslike. "Tell me, why the interest in this flour sample?"

"I'm trying to track its progress from a field in America to a destination in Africa."

"Ah." She studied her glass. She did not look mouselike any more. "Why?"

"Curiosity," I said. "With reference to a series of events in the Third World."

She said, "I shouldn't . . . I can't really help. I mean, it's only a rumor."

I said, "I'm a poet, not a scientist. My rules of evidence are pretty slack."

She smiled uneasily, took a heartening sip of wine. She said, "I took the liberty . . . I, er, had a research student follow up the literature." She was looking very nervous now.

I said, "What do you mean?"

She said, "It's not a big field. I mean, not many grain producers feel the need to mark their produce. So I thought . . . well, this afternoon I had my student make a search of the appropriate publications. We found four specialists. I made inquiries. And we found one experiment last year in the Midwest."

I said, "Go slower."

She smiled. She was getting confident again. "It was a most interesting exercise," she said. "And I think we found who marked your corn."

I stared at her.

"I can't tell you the scientist's name," she said. "But I can tell you the farmer."

I said, "Wonderful."

"It was in Ohio. Somewhere near Cleveland. His name"— her eyes flicked left and right. John was knotting string in the corner, next to an orange juice—"was Bruno Wanamaker. The isotope was the one in your sample. It could be a coincidence, but it's very unlikely. Er . . . I'd rather this went no further."

I said, "Of course not." I finished the wine, stood up. "I'm very grateful to you," I said.

"I never said a word." There was actual fright behind the smile, as if she had done something she now regretted. "Particularly not if you're talking to Charis. Charis is very . . . formal. Very discreet." Then she remembered herself. "So anyway. Thank you for the reading. It was just beautiful." Her eyelashes were trembling over her eyes. I kissed her on the cheek. I found I was thinking of Ricky Lee. John was looking pointedly in the other direction. We left.

In the Mustang, John said, "She's after your body, man."

"Never mind that," I said. I was still thinking of Ricky Lee. "We're going to Cleveland."

I could not face the drive back to Quogue, so we checked into a motel by the airport. I shut myself into my cabin, and called information. There was only one Bruno Wanamaker in Ohio. He lived near Ganges, a good stretch southwest of Cleveland. I called Bethel Bay. There was no reply. So I wrote a letter to the boys. Sinsemilla fumes began to filter through the ventilator from next door, mixed with the lurch and clank of the Grateful Dead.

Next morning, the motel courtesy bus took us to the airport, and we caught the 10:44 Continental flight to Cleveland.

I swallowed my heart, which as usual when I was flying was in my mouth, and gave myself over to prayer. John drank four beers and gazed with frank interest at the landscape sliding under the window. He was wearing his bodyguard uniform, but with a skull-and-roses T-shirt instead of the white nylon shirt. He had retained the leather tie. I closed my eyes while the pilot slammed the plane on to the runway. By the time we had secured a hire car and pointed the nose southwest, the time was four o'clock.

We moved out into a country of barns and silos. The barns were painted oxide-red and copper-green. Some of the buildings looked faded, beginning to peel. But the wheat fields were neat, brilliant squares of green, tinged with the blue of plenty of nitrogen fertilizer. At six o'clock, we arrived.

Bruno Wanamaker lived in a square wooden house, painted iron-oxide red with white windows. The house sat in the exact center of an expanse of mown green grass, with two symmetrically placed maples and a white picket fence. The green grass sat in the middle of four L-shaped paddocks. There were three elegant chestnut horses in one of the paddocks. Beyond the paddocks to the east of the house was a barn, the hipped roof tiled with cedar shingles weathered to a soft silver. The sky was blue, without a trace of haze. A fat stormcloud lay across the eastern horizon. The westering sun showed every wrinkle and bulge of the cloud, just as you could see every ridge and gully in the corrugated iron cladding of the conglomeration of huge sheds and silos beyond the wooden barn.

"Toytown," said John.

It was toytown, if you ignored the steel buildings. If you took the buildings into account, it was a fair-sized factory. I drove up the perfect blacktop drive to the back of the house and parked next to two pickups and a Lincoln Continental. John fitted in like a steel desk in a cabinetmaker's workshop. I said, "Stay in the car." He pulled the inevitable length of string out of the pocket of the golf jacket and began to knot. I walked across the blacktop and rang the doorbell.

A woman opened it. She had a gray face, glasses, colorless hair worn long in a style that was too young for her. She was wearing a white blouse with a collar like the frill on a lamb cutlet and a straight black skirt that came down to her knees. She looked efficient but unwelcoming. I said, "Is Mr. Wanamaker still here?"

She gave me a confidential secretary's once-over. "I don't believe he's expecting you," she said. What she was seeing was a medium-sized, thinnish man wearing an acceptable jacket and tie, with hair that needed cutting and an English accent. She frowned. She said, "Have I seen you somewhere?"

I said, "On TV, maybe?"

She frowned again, then a tide of pink rose out of the frill and lapped at her hairline. "Oh!" she said. "Sure. I saw you on News Actuality, right? You're the guy who had the problems with the boat? And the Ethiopia story?" She put out her hand. I shook it. She was sweating with enthusiasm. "Wait a minute," she said, recollecting herself. "You're not . . . soliciting donations?"

"Not soliciting," I said, with as close as I could manage to a TV personality grin. "I just need to talk to Mr. Wanamaker."

She said, "That's good," as if she meant it. "Come on in."

Bruno Wanamaker was a small puce man with wispy hair that was blond going on gray. He was sitting in a hide swiveler at a desk with a computer, a stock screen, and a complicated telephone. He was wearing a leather jacket and Gucci loafers. On the wall was a calendar from the Moorings Beach Club, Antigua, and a photograph of a gray gunboat, vintage WWII, with a younger, hairier Wanamaker grinning on the bridge. I did not know much about American farmers, but he looked a good deal more cosmopolitan than your straight-down-the-line Eastern Midwestern hayseed. His secretary said, "This is Mr. Devis."

His eyes were muddy blue and watchful. His smile missed them by several hundred yards. "Devis," he said. "Any kin to old Dandy Devis?"

"I'm English," I said.

"So's Dandy," he said, and grinned, as if he had scored points. "Now what can we do for you?"

I said, "It's rather a tricky business."

He said, "I guess you aren't selling anything, looking the way you do, arriving this late in the day. So spit it out."

I said, "You grow wheat, right?"

He said, "Like my old petty officer used to say, does a bear shit in the woods?"

I smiled, trying to look as if it was a new one. "Within the last couple of years, you sold a consignment for shipment to Ethiopia."

He shrugged. He said, "We grow twenty-five thousand tons a year. As long as the price is right, who cares where it goes?"

"Of course," I said. Had the eyes become a fraction more watchful? "But part of that load was . . . special."

"Wheat's wheat," he said. Again there was the grin, as if he had scored points.

"Someone turned up here and asked you to spray an acreage with a radioactive isotope of iodine," I said. "That's what made it special."

The eyes were definitely watchful now. He said, "What makes you think that?"

"I was told."

"Then you either believe what you were told, or you don't."

He smiled. "I just don't see any way I can help you." His face was not fat. It was round, but hard as pink granite. It was the face of a man who had been turning land into money ever since he had left the U.S. Navy.

I said, "I'm trying to trace this consignment. It could be linked to a major crime. Double murder."

He said, "Are you a policeman?"

I said, "My sister was one of the people murdered."

He arched his eyebrows on his pink forehead. "Fascinating story," he said. "Sorry about your sister. I will tell you that this marking was done after representations made to me by a shipping agent, after a request made to them by a government agency."

Aid and spooks, I thought. How do you get into a government agency? "Which one?" I said.

He smiled. He was going to talk about himself now. "Sir, I am a good Republican," he said. "I do not know and I do not care. All I know is that Less Government is Better Government. I am sitting here watching a wheat price that is giving me stomach acid. They paid me five thousand dollars over and above what I was paid for the corn. Let me tell you that with farming the way it is around here, five thousand dollars is not something you turn down. No siree." The glow went out as if he had flicked a switch. I thought of the farmers of the village, with their mud granaries and their implements made with endless labor from the leaf-springs of old trucks. Esias would have been very polite about Mr. Wanamaker, and thought his own thoughts. Camilla would have smiled sweetly, and made him do what she wanted him to do.

Personally, I stood there and nodded sympathetically, and said, "Times are hard all over," and hoped I would not be struck by lightning.

Wanamaker said, "Well, that's all I can tell you. I'm sure you have other appointments." He turned his swivel chair to the desk and started to tap the keyboard in front of his screen.

I said, "Thank you for your help." He nodded, absently. I showed myself out.

The secretary was waiting in the outside office, smiling anxiously. She said, "I heard on the intercom. I'm real sorry. Bruno . . . he's not always like this. It's just that wheat's real bad right now, and it's the end of the day . . . the week . . ."

I wiped the sweat of anger from my palms on the lining of my coat pockets. I said, "I understand." The poor woman was wringing her hands. Oh, the magic of television. "I just needed to find out the name of the shipping agent, that's all."

She glanced over her shoulder. "Listen," she said in a half-whisper. "I remember that consignment. It was smaller than usual. It went to J. J. Birdman in Cleveland." She glanced at the door. Wanamaker was talking loudly about money into his fancy telephone. She opened a filing cabinet, consulted a computer printout. "Consignment number," she said, scribbling on a piece of paper. She gave me the paper, put her finger to her lips, eyebrows up by her hairline. "He works too hard," she said. "He's a very kind man, really."

I folded the paper into my pocket. "It's been really nice to meet you," I said.

"And you," she said. Her voice was fluttering like a damaged bird. "Good *luck*," she whispered, squeezing my hand.

Scotch John was finishing off a complicated knob knot on his lanyard. He said, "That was fast."

I pulled the car's nose down the driveway and out on to the road. I said, "Have you ever met any FBI agents?"

"I seen some DEA."

"DEA?"

"Drug Enforcement Administration. Federal."

"That'll do. Can you behave like one?"

John nodded his big head slowly. "I kin issue threats and beat the shit out of folks."

"Not that level of enforcement."

"Excuse me, sir," said John. "I have here a warrant to search this car for substances I have reason to believe contravene federal ordinances pertaining to transportation of narcotics across a state line."

"That's fine," I said.

"Where are we going?"

"Motel," I said. "Then Cleveland, to see some corn shippers. On behalf of your new employers, the government of the United States of America."

19

NEXT MORNING, JOHN DROVE WHILE I SQUINTED AT THE MAP.
People were milling around clapboard churches, wearing stiff
suits and hats. We found an open clothing store and stopped
outside. I told John to buy an FBI rig-out while I found a public
telephone and called Birdman's. A nasal voice told me they
were open, unloading a ship. John emerged from the store
wearing a pea green anorak, an Oxford stripe shirt, and a pair
of polyester slacks, maroon. The burst-sofa hair was yanked
back in a ponytail and the eyes were hidden behind a pair of
RayBans. "Behold the G-man from Hell," he said.

As he drove on, I told him what he had to do. "Yeah," he
said. "I like this better than bodyguarding."

By late morning, Cleveland was extending grubby concrete
arms to fold us in. It was eleven-thirty by the time we arrived at
the lakeshore. There was a long chainlink fence with a high
steel gate, open. Inside the gate was a wharf. There was a ship
alongside, big and black, with the bridge at the top of a lump of
superstructure at its forward end. Proximity to water seemed to
have perked John up. "Laker," he said. "Bridge forward, so he
can see where he's going."

J. J. Birdman was a tall iron grain elevator alongside the wharf. At the foot of the elevator was a flat-roofed building with plate-glass windows, dwarfed by the monstrous height of the blank iron walls above. One of its doors said OFFICE. Trucks were waiting under the elevator, augers like the probosces of insects sucking grain from their trailers.

We left the car by the trucks. I let John lead the way through the door.

There was a counter painted chipped green. The battered man behind it looked up from his newspaper. "Yeah?" he said.

John said, "I need to talk to the boss."

The man reeked of old cigarettes. I could smell him from where I was standing, hands in jacket pockets by the door. "Who you?" he said.

"Government business," said John. "Where's Mr. Birdman?"

"Dead forty years," he said. "You want Mr. Cullis."

John said, "Yeah."

The man said, "Do you have an appointment?"

John was leaning on the counter, fingers twined. His hands looked like four pounds of country pork sausages. He glanced at me sideways, and said, "We request your cooperation in this matter."

"Who are you?" said the man doggedly.

"Mr. Cullis may tell you, after we are through," said John. "Now do you call him, or do I come through and fetch him?"

The battered man looked at John. John looked back. The battered man's hand shook slightly as he lit a cigarette. He lifted the telephone and said, "Mr. Cullis? Couple guys here say they're from the govmint." He put back the receiver. "He says come on in," he said.

John turned his head toward me. "Agent Fester?" he said. I followed him through the office, up some steps and into a room with a carpet and a bald man.

The bald man smiled hospitably and gave us chairs. He said, "How can I help you?"

This was where John had to stop improvising and work to script. He stuck out his legs, tucked in his chin. He said, "CIA/FBI joint investigation. Internal audit. Division of responsibility, job description. I have here a consignment number, authorized by my department. I need to know for confirmation purposes the identity of the consignee."

The bald man said, "Do you have ID?" The obliging smile did not flicker. The eyes did, measuring John up and down. Corn shippers knew about aid. Aid and spooks.

John pulled out my wallet, extracted my British Library reader's card. He moved close to the bald man, so the bald man could see, if he had not seen already, that if he stood up, his nose would arrive only at the base of John's sternum. The bald man could not concentrate on the ID. The skin of his cranium took on a pasty gleam.

"Now," said John. "Please furnish Agent Fester with the information I have requested."

The bald man's smile turned nervous. "Sure," he said. "Of course. Right now. Just give me the consignment number."

I stepped forward. John stepped back, handing over to his subordinate. "I'll be in the car," he said. "Call to make." It was a bodyguard move: cover the entrance.

I wrote down the consignment number Wanamaker's secretary had given me. The bald man battered keys on his computer. He said, "Date November last. Consignee, Aid Services, Port Sudan. Consignor's name, Emergency Relief Bureau." He smiled. "But you already know that."

I kept my face still. I nodded and wrote down the particulars in a spiral-bound notebook. I said, "Thank you for your cooperation."

"Any time," he said.

I clattered down the stairs. Out on the concrete where the trucks were parked, someone was yelling. I could hear the noise as I went through the outer office, but not the words. I opened the door.

There was the roar of the wind off the lake, the grind of a big truck warming up its diesel. And over the top of it, a man's voice. *"All right, you son of a bitch,"* it was yelling, *"move right on over."*

John's voice. He was standing by the car, big as a house in his pea green anorak, his beard whipping in the wind off the lake. Opposite him, with their backs to me, were two men with wide shoulders. One was black, the other was white.

They did not look around. The office door slammed behind me. The white one of the duo turned. He had long, flat cheeks and cheekbones like the eye protectors on a boxer's sparring helmet. My stomach was suddenly hollow, my mouth dry.

The face was familiar. I had seen it in Quogue harbor and on Ellerton Street in Cambridge. It was the face of whoever had come aboard *Halcyon* and stolen the urn full of flour.

John said, "They were trying to get in the car."

The black man aimed a punch at John. John put his arm up to block it. The black man did something else that looked professional and very fast. John said, *"Oof."* He bent double. The black man kicked him. John fell over. There was a loud, nasty *crack* as his head hit the concrete. He did not get up.

I did not believe it was happening.

It was happening, all right.

The white man had gnarled, stubby fingers that flexed and unflexed at the ends of the sleeves of his baseball jacket. Under the jacket, the black fist T-shirt crawled over the muscles of the chest. His face did not move. He walked toward me, casually, not in a hurry.

My knees were showing a tendency to knock. I shouted, "Police!" Behind me, the door stayed shut, and the window. "Police!" I yelled again.

"Shaddap," said the white man. His mouth did not shape the word. A slot opened and the syllables fell out. He came on like a landslide.

My throat was full of sand, and the bottom had dropped out of my stomach.

I could see what he wanted in the boneless nose, the killer

eyeslits, the lips smashed back over the teeth. He wanted to hurt. I already knew he knew how. I did not know why.

I ran anyway.

One moment, I was standing there. The next I was moving away from the gate, past the elevator, my legs going like pistons. Behind me, someone was shouting. Engines were roaring, and the wind was wailing off the lake. I ran into the wind like a rabbit. I went past the office. There was a face at the window. I yelled, but I could not tell if any sound came out. My foot skidded on a brown iron rail set in the paving. I was on the quay, heading for the tall black side of the ship tied up alongside. To the right, the buildings went as far as the water's edge. To the left was a strip of open quay bounded on its inland side by the grain elevator and on the lake side by the black iron hull of the ship.

I turned left. I could hear the thump of the boxer's sneakers. He was too heavy to be fast. All right, I thought, I'll keep my distance until the police arrive. I ran on, along the strip of quay between the ship's side and the grain elevator. I thought: Once I get out the other end, he will never catch me.

Ahead, a figure moved into the gap. It was a thickset figure, tall, with wide, sloping shoulders. It was the black man who had knocked down Scotch John.

To my left, the grain elevator was a black iron cliff. An iron cliff with a ladder up the side. There were galleries above.

The footsteps behind me were easy and relaxed, the footsteps of a man used to workouts in the gym, and trackwork, and whacking people's heads off. I could still hear the *clonk* as John's head hit the ground.

I hated ladders. But the ladder was the best there was.

I slapped my hands on the iron rungs and began to climb.

I climbed quickly, the way you go up the rigging of a boat, weight out, feet and hands moving in fast sequence. I did not mind climbing. It was what happened when you got to the top that I minded.

I was breathing hard now. The sweat was running. Through

the rungs of the ladder I could feel the vibration of other feet and hands. The iron wall flowed past. I did not want to look down.

But I had to.

I turned my head. The sides of the ladder converged sharply toward the pale, upturned face of the boxer. Below the boxer, a parked jeep was the size of a toy. My knees turned to string. The boxer's mouth widened in a letterbox smile. It was the height that was the problem, not the smile. Vertigo, I thought. I started to howl. Vertigo.

My hands were skipping on the iron. I was fit, but not as fit as a boxer. Tiredness was making me ragged. I looked up.

Fifteen feet above my head, the ladder went through a hole in the gallery. Above the gallery, the iron side of the elevator swept up another fifty feet to the rim. The sky was rushing past up there, so the elevator reeled against the clouds. My head began to swim again. I thrust my head and shoulders through the hole, scrambled on to the grill.

Right, you bastard, I thought. This is where I take you as you come through the hole.

Then I thought of a fight up here, seventy feet above the quay. Me, trained by Camilla's old boyfriend for a weekend on a cottage lawn. Him, a professional boxer. The gallery's handrail was a single iron bar, supported every ten feet. It would be dead easy to fall through, plummet into space.

My knees dissolved again. I lurched to the inside of the catwalk, put my hand on the comforting iron wall of the elevator, began to shuffle along the wall like a drunk.

A couple of hundred feet of steel gallery away, the black man heaved his shoulders through another hole in the catwalk. I heard the thump and ring of feet close behind me. A voice said, "You *daid*."

There was a door. It was a steel door, set flush in the wall of the elevator. I leaped at the door, wrenched at the handle. It opened. I charged through, slammed it, looked for a bolt. There was no bolt. There was a keyhole, but no key in it.

My eyes were adjusting to the gloom.

I was on a gallery, twin to the one outside, except that this one was under cover. It ran along the side of a row of giant bins. There was the heavy smell of bulk grain. The air was dim, hazy with corn dust. I heard a door open behind me, then slam shut. The sound roared in the steel cave. I started to run forward. The breath was wheezing in my throat. A shaft of light lanced across the gallery ahead as another door opened. Spotlit in the glare stood the black boxer. I could see the sun gleaming in the gold rings on his hands.

He stopped. The footsteps behind me stopped. I stopped. There were no more doors.

There was a boxer at either end. There was a straight run of metal gallery, bordered on the one side by a steel wall with machinery, and on the other by the line of grain bins.

High above, I could hear the twitter of sparrows. There would be a good living for a sparrow in here. The dust was irritating my throat. I could hear my breathing, loud and hot, harsh in my skull.

The black man said, "You got to slow down. You got to take it easy." His voice caught tinny echoes from the roof.

The white man said, "We going to hurt you."

The black man said, "They tell us not to kill you. They tell us to hurt you."

The white man said, "To hurt you so you wish you *daid*."

The black man said, "Hurt you *bad*."

The white man said, "Because you asking too many *questions*."

The black man said, "And questions is nothing but *trouble*."

The door was still open. I saw the sun gleam on his white teeth as he smiled. "And if you ask any more questions," he said, "you could *die*."

"Die *daid*," said the white man.

The black man shut the door. In the gloom, he looked huge; even bigger than the white man. "Ready, Jackson?" he said.

Jackson hitched up the sleeves of his coat, settled his head into his big shoulders. "Ready, Gerard."

One from each end, slow as afternoon strollers, they started toward me.

I looked at the bins.

They were filled with shadow. Beneath the shadow was the pale golden light of the wheat twenty feet down. I was standing at the place where one bin butted up against its neighbor. The top of the wall that separated them was six inches wide. It went across the width of the building, forty feet to another catwalk on the far side.

The parapet was three feet high. I pulled myself on to the top of it and began to walk across.

Twenty feet below, the corn gleamed like sand dunes. The bins were hoppers, like giant funnels. Lorries parked under them to be loaded. I walked slow and careful, like a tightrope walker, one foot in front of the other.

Gerard said, "Shoot him."

You bloody fool, I thought. This is America, where people carry guns. No, I told myself. They're not here to kill me. They said they weren't.

My body did not believe me. My back crawled as I walked along the narrow wall. Waiting for the bullet.

Somewhere behind me, there was an enormous explosion. I jumped convulsively. I was halfway along the wall. I staggered, tried to regain my balance.

I fell.

20

I SLAMMED INTO THE CORN FLAT ON MY BACK. THE AIR WHOOSHED out of me. I was gasping like a goldfish, head ringing, sliding down a slope of grain. There was a lot of pain and trying to breathe. Somewhere underneath that was the idea of an ant slithering into the funnel of an ant-lion hole. The slithering stopped. I got a breath, full of the mealy taste of dust. I got another.

I was lying on my back in the base of the funnel-shaped depression that had formed when someone had let corn out of the hopper. It was almost a comfortable place to lie, except for the dust in the lungs, and the pain in the back, and the fear.

And the noise.

The high vault of the roof was full of the noise. It sounded like the yell of a peacock, grossly amplified. Not a peacock. A kookaburra.

Jackson and Gerard were laughing.

I rolled on to my hands and knees. The hands sank into the corn. The fear was turning to anger. Dial-a-heavy, I thought. Mr. Sullivan and Mr. Wanamaker had made their calls. When I get out of here, I am going to find out who had been on the other end.

If you get out of here.

When, said the anger. Laugh on, you bastards. I looked up. There were two heads up there. One of them waved an arm.

On the far side of the corn bin I could see a series of short horizontal lines, parallel to each other, extending from the surface of the corn up the side of the bin. Ladder rungs. A way out.

The heads disappeared.

I started up the side of the funnel-shaped depression in the corn. Laughter was still whanging around the roof girders. Somewhere in the shed I heard a *clunk,* the whine of a motor.

Over the whine of the motor there was another sound: a gentle, slipping hiss.

The sheet of corn up which I was climbing began to move. I knew why they were laughing.

The faster I climbed, the faster the corn seemed to slide. Dust was rising out of the sides of the funnel like cigarette smoke from a football crowd. It stuck in the sweat and itched. The breath wheezed in the lungs. There was worse than itching. My hands and feet had disappeared beneath the surface. The grains were shifting down there, slipping one over the other.

There were new noises above the whining, far away, in another world. It was a safe world. It was not very far away, but it might as well have been at the other end of the universe. Police sirens were wailing. Somewhere or other, I heard the slap of training shoes on a catwalk. I could not see anything beyond the dust except a high, dark vault of girders and a pale slope of corn running up to the dark edge of the bin. Part of the pale slope detached itself from the rest. It rolled down and slapped me in the face.

The slope became suddenly fluid. I lost my arms and legs completely. I got a gulp of dust and air. The grain flowed over me, or I sank into the grain, I could not tell which. It was all over me, like liquid, except you can swim in liquid.

I had the picture of a world full of fluid corn, and a body in the center of it, and in the center of the body a mind, and in the mind a single thought.

Don't breathe.

Everything was turning red, blood color. There was a leather strap around my chest and springs of panic trying to uncoil against it, saying *breathe.* But the part of the mind, the seat of the will, kept nagging through the crescendo roar of blood in the ears.

Don't breathe.

I thrashed like a dying fish. The corn hindered my movements. My right hand was suddenly cold. Cold meant something.

Air.

I rolled toward my right hand.

My face was in air. I breathed, floundered, rolled again. The corn had become solid. I found more air. The whine of the motor had gone. Gingerly, I moved a leg. A layer of corn slid sullenly, stopped. I moved an arm. I coughed. The surface stayed still. I lay there and breathed. The air was full of dust, but it tasted better than Swiss sanatorium breezes. The warm oxygen spread to arms and legs and brain. Slowly, I began to crawl up the slope to the rungs set in the side of the bin.

The corn shifted. I moved slowly, half-climbing, half-swimming, up the down escalator, two feet forward, one foot back. Sweat carved channels through the dust on my face.

When I got to the bottom rung I hooked my fingers over it, laid my head on the corn slope, and closed my eyes. I felt as if I had run fifteen miles in mud. Move, said the mind. Keep going. I pulled myself up, groped for the bottom rung with my toes, and hauled myself above the surface. The sirens were still wailing out there. I climbed. I heaved myself over the parapet of the bin.

I had finally made it across the elevator. There was a catwalk, a mirror image of the other side. I leaned against the steel wall and coughed dust back into the bin. My mind began to work.

I walked along the catwalk to a door, opened it a crack, and peered out.

Down below was the yard, with the offices and a couple of trucks. There was an ambulance in the yard, and a police car. The police car's lights were flashing like electric strawberries. The policemen were leaning against it, talking to Mr. Cullis. It would have been Mr. Cullis who had called the police. Which meant that Jackson and Gerard were not known to Mr. Cullis. Furthermore, Jackson and Gerard would not have had time to go over my car, if the tape was what they were after. Mr. Cullis was shrugging his shoulders. He looked as if he was saying that he had no shred or trace of a goddamn clue what was happening, there was this FBI guy, and some guys who knocked over this other guy right there in the yard, and those guys like vanished, and was the job of the Police Department not to protect honest businesspersons such as himself against such sonsabitches? Mr. Cullis was waving his arms a lot. He did not look pleased. There was no sign of Jackson and Gerard. The policemen drew their pistols and went for the end of the elevator, where I had seen a door that probably led to some stairs.

I stood there for a moment, peering through the crack high above the yard, itching with sweat and grain dust.

The ambulance must be for John. Mr. Cullis would have told the FBI story. When the police got to him in the hospital and found that he had identified himself with my British Library reader's card, they would certainly check his bona fides and mine. I had no idea what the penalties were for impersonating Secret Service agents. I had no desire to find out. I walked quickly down the catwalk to the opposite end from the one at which the police had come in. There was a flight of stairs here as well. I scuttled down it, opened the door. Mr. Cullis had his back to me. I ran hard across the yard. My lungs were wheezing thickly. I opened the car door, started the engine and stamped on the throttle. Mr. Cullis's face looked white and stretched.

I could see why. There were nozzles in the side of the

elevator, designed to fill trucks with wheat. Underneath one of the nozzles was a huge golden pyramid of corn with a truck half-buried in it.

I could hear Jackson and Gerard. *We going to hurt you bad. If you ask any more questions, you could die.*

They had turned on the corn and watched me sink. Then they had turned off the corn.

Kind of them.

I jumped into the car, twisted the key and mashed the throttle into the floorboards. At the gate, I hauled the wheel over, screeched into the main road, turned right behind the billboard that masked the elevator from the highway. Unless Mr. Cullis had eyes like an osprey, he would not have been able to read the number plate.

After half a mile I began to shake so badly that I could not keep my foot on the accelerator. I hauled the car into the parking lot of a Burger King by the lakeshore and sat and stared at the gray-blue shift of Lake Erie, waiting for the shuddering to go away.

You are not dead, I said to myself. Unlike Rhyd and Camilla, you are not dead.

I found I could think about what I had to do next. The shaking went. I was feeling cold and sick.

I climbed out of the car and slapped at my clothes. A cloud of corn dust billowed into the wind, floated inland across Lake Shore Boulevard back toward the farms it had come from. Through the corn dust I could taste the flat, chemical whiff of a big body of polluted water.

I beat out more dust. A couple of ring-billed gulls were riding the wind above the lake, waiting for things to wash up on the beach. I could have been one of those things.

A voice behind me said, "George."

My heart jumped into my mouth and my stomach vanished. I turned around, hands bunching. I was looking at a woman wearing jeans and a T-shirt that flapped in the breeze off the lake. She had reddish hair and eyes set in an awkward slant in her head.

I tried to say, "Ricky Lee." For a second, I felt a relief that was like a homecoming. Then I woke up. I said, "What the hell?"

She said, "Bill got as far as Birdman's. Then he got stuck."

I put my hands on the car roof and laid my head on them and closed my eyes. It was quiet, and dark, and it soothed the throb in my head and the hot ache in my upper chest.

I felt a hand on my shoulder. Ricky Lee said, "You need coffee."

The idea that coffee could even dent my present condition was hilarious. The fingers tugged. I moved.

She said, "I'll order. Get into the washroom." She shoved a small mauve hairbrush into my hand. It was a strangely intimate gesture. Then I realized it could be a gesture of authority, not intimacy. Like all good reporters I have ever met, she gave the impression that she was following an excellent mental map all of her own. Fuzzily, I thought: All that stuff earlier on, the flake-gets-a-break stuff. Wool over the eyes, Devis. All along.

Or maybe that was what having a steady job on the *Echo* did for you.

I propped myself up against the washbasin and cleaned myself. I used the hairbrush. I turned from a gray-haired red-eyed poet into a brown-haired red-eyed poet. The eyes looked sunken, as if in shock or near death. A silt of questions began to accumulate in my mind, burying the moment of intimacy.

When I went back she was sitting in a blind corner, away from the window, bolt upright, mouth set hard. She said, "I bought you coffee. What happened?"

I ignored her. I said, "How did you get here?"

She stared at me. She opened her mouth. She looked as if she was going to say something angry. Then she seemed to see something in my face that persuaded her this would not be a good idea.

I said, "You found John and me here. How?"

She raised her eyebrows. "Just as goddamn well I did," she said.

"How?"

She dropped her eyes and fiddled with her plastic coffee spoon.

"Tell me the truth," I said.

"I was making inquiries."

"Rubbish," I said. She raised her eyes. They were hard, talk-if-you-dare eyes. "I went to see Sullivan. You were the only person who knew I was going. A guy in a fist shirt was waiting for me when I came out of the house. He tried to cave my ribs in. And there he was again today, warning me off, and here you are again today. I think we should go to your new editor and ask him if he thinks you are reporting this story or whether you are part of this story."

She was very pale. She said, "No."

I said, "Why not?"

She said, "I was holding out on you."

I was tired. I leaned into the angle the wall made with the plastic banquette. I said, "What does that mean?"

She put her hands on the table. The left hand had the fingernails cut short: guitar player's fingernails on a journalist. "I went down to argue with Sullivan," she said. "You'd just been. He was angry, scared, I dunno. It was six A.M., but he was halfway in the bag. So I, like, made myself pleasant." She was getting into the story now. She had made her lips look softer and the humor was back in the slanted eyes. I was thinking of us as friends again. I remembered how much she had been in my mind lately. If this was the stuff she had used on Sullivan, Sullivan would not have had a chance. "So I gave him a ride to the airport, him and his fishing rods, and I bought him some margaritas for breakfast, and I got him to talk about Bill. He had no idea what story Bill was on, which was fine, because as you know Bill did not tell people things, least of all his editor. But he started in talking about expenses claims. And I guessed that you were on the same story as Bill. I went to the *Echo* and took his expenses claims off the computer. And I called Pierce Rapaport, and he said you were in Portland. But you weren't at Quogue, and nor was John. So I called a friend at the airport, and she got into the system and told me you were on a flight to Cleveland. And I found a ticket to Cleveland on Bill's expenses for January this year. And I found this, in my book." She laid a notebook on the table.

It was a black notebook with an elastic band marking the page. The page was numbered with a date stamp that read *Jan. 4.* There were scribbled notes, in a hand I recognized as hers. There was the name J. J. Birdman, and two numbers. One of them was a telephone number. The other was a meaningless string of digits.

Except that it was not meaningless, because it was the consignment number of Bruno Wanamaker's shipment of irradiated wheat, dispatched by J. J. Birdman to Aid Services of Port Sudan.

"He dictated those down the phone before he went to Africa," she said. "So I guessed you might go to Birdman's, too. So I . . . pulled a little stakeout."

"And the guys in the shirts were nothing to do with you."

Her eyes narrowed. She said, "What are you talking about?" She sounded angry and disappointed.

"One of them burgled the boat. He found me at Sullivan's. He found me today."

"So Sullivan called him. So someone called him the other times. You think I did it? Listen, buster. I want this story. But you're part of it, right? Why would I get someone to beat up on you?"

I drank coffee. She asked if I wanted a donut. I tried not to believe her. It was no good. My brain might be full of corn dust, but I believed her, all right.

I said, "So who are those people?"

"People?"

"A black man and a white man. Big." I told her what had happened at the elevator.

She said, "I was by the gate, in the car. I saw them arrive, I saw them leave. I saw their faces."

I said, "They are interested in the same things I'm interested in."

"*We're* interested in."

"Of course."

She sipped coffee. She said. "They're professional fighters."

I said, wearily, "I know."

She said, "Those shirts."

"What about them?"

" 'Warren's,' " she said. "Black fist in a glove. That's the logo."

"Warren's?"

"Fight gym. South Boston. Belongs to a guy called Warren Diglis."

I stared at her.

She said, "What's the problem?"

I said, "I've met Mr. Diglis."

Warren Diglis had called me a white imperialist. I remembered what he had said after the speech at the Cambridge Regency. *Now you look after yourself, you hear?*

Or he would do the looking after.

"Bad guy," she said. "Politically acceptable armed robber. Why?"

I said, "He thinks he's a friend of Ras Hamil."

She raised her eyebrows. "How do you know?"

"He told me." I was after Ras Hamil's blood. It would not be surprising if he was after mine, or doing his best to frighten me away.

I said, "We should find John."

"The guy in the ambulance said Sacred Heart Hospital."

I was worried about what could be happening at the Sacred Heart Hospital. I told her what I wanted her to do. She made a face. I said, "Do you know Cleveland?"

"I was on a student attachment with the *Plain Dealer*," she said. She laughed. "One of the many. You can follow me."

I tailed her yellow Chevrolet through the beginning of the rush hour.

Sullivan called Jackson down on me. Farmer Bruno Wanamaker had called in Jackson and Gerard, or someone who controlled them. I did not believe Jackson and Gerard were working for Ras Hamil. I believed they were working for the Emergency Resources Bureau. Which was an arm of the U.S. Government. But if Warren Diglis and Ras Hamil had things in common, that meant that Hamil and the U.S. Government had Diglis in common.

I did not understand.

A coldness raised goose pimples on my spine. There was one central issue.

Whoever they were working for, Jackson and Gerard had warned me off with a promise of worse next time.

It was hard to imagine worse than what had happened at J. J. Birdman, in the corn . . .

I said, "Bloody hell."

Ricky Lee made a right. I cut across a stream of traffic in a blare of horns, hanging on to the wheel with one hand, clattering in the glovebox with the other. I found the Sullivan cassette, shoved it in the slot, rewound it. The yellow Chevrolet dived left. There was the guitar, Rhyd's voice:

> It's worse than that there, Elmer,
> There's a birdman in the corn.

I started to rewind the tape. Ricky Lee pulled over to the curb. I pulled the tape out, shoved it in my pocket. I walked along to her window, told her what I wanted her to do. She said, "Is this a good idea?"

"Up to you," I said. "You're the bait."

She smiled. "The story," she said. *"Toujours* the story." She patted my hand, left hers on mine. It felt about right there. "Be careful."

"Of course," I said.

There was a thick silence. She noticed where her hand was.

She blushed, climbed into my passenger seat. We drove two blocks to the hospital.

The hospital smelled cool and clean. I had a great urge to lie down on the floor and press my forehead against the cool tiles. I said, "Let's find out where he is."

She smiled at me. I watched her walk across the floor. I had forgotten her dancer's walk. In her big T-shirt, she looked like any of the other nice girls who were strolling Cleveland this free-as-air day in early summer. She needed to be looked at, to draw away the eyes of anyone who would be looking out for George Devis.

She came back, faster than she had gone. "He has a concussion," she said, louder than was necessary. Then, quieter: "There's a cop with him. He's in B15."

I said, loud, "Wait here. I'm going to see the bastard."

Her odd-slanting eyes widened in protest. Her mouth opened, registering anger. She was a good actress. Before she could speak, I said, "If you don't want me to talk to that slimeball, you come right along up and stop me."

There were a dozen people in a waiting room off the reception area. A few eyes shifted in our direction, drawn by the whiff of aggravation.

Ricky Lee's teeth came together with a click. "Thank *you*," she said. "He can look after himself, and you. I'll wait down here. He's in B15." She stuck a hand on her hip. "Careful he don't eat you up, now."

I said, "I'll be right down."

21

I WALKED UP THE VINYL STAIRS. NOBODY EVEN GLANCED AT ME. B15 was on the first floor. I waited in the corner of the corridor, looking for hovering policemen. There were none. I walked quickly past 12, 13, 14. Fifteen had a glass panel in the door. Through the panel I saw John, lying in bed. His head was bandaged, his beard spread out over the sheet. His eyes were half-closed. There was a man sitting by the side of the bed, reading what looked like a volume of Reader's Digest condensed books. He had short hair and a leathery face. He looked more like a cop than a doctor. John's eyes were on the glass panel. He saw my face. He closed the eye furthest from the policeman in a slow, discreet wink.

I waved. I walked back down the corridor to the internal telephone. I got the number of the room from reception; dialed. A voice said, "Hello?"

I said, "Lieutenant Murray to see you in reception, sir." I did my best to sound American.

The voice said, "Who's Lieutenant Murray?"

I said, "He's standing right here, sir. He says will you please step down?"

The voice said, "I'm on guard duty here. I don't know no Lieutenant Murray."

I was beginning to sweat. I said, "Lieutenant Murray says he, er, I don't like to tell you what he says. Excuse me." I covered the mouthpiece with my hand, made a buzzing noise. "He says either you get down here or he will bust your ass."

"Tell him—"

I hung up. My palms were slippery. I walked away around a corner and stood in front of the bank of elevators. After a couple of minutes I heard the door open and ill-tempered feet clump down the corridor. As soon as he was out of sight I walked quickly back and opened the door. "John," I said.

He sat up in bed. He was wearing blue striped hospital pajamas. He grabbed his head.

"Do you want to stay in?" I said.

He winked alternate eyes, experimenting. "Jesus no," he said. "They haven't found your card yet, but they took my clothes."

"Quick," I said.

He picked up his head like a Ming bowl, lurched across the floor. "Ooh," he said. "Hurts." I opened the door for him. We went off down the corridor toward the elevators. He was zigzagging badly. Someone had left a wheelchair in the corridor. I stabbed the elevator button and said, "Sit down." He sat, groaning. He only just fitted between the arms.

The ward next door was empty. I twitched two blankets off the bed, shoved one around his knees and one over his head. He looked like a huge, bearded Russian grandmother, easily weird enough to stop people asking questions out of simple pity. The elevator arrived. I pushed him in. The elevator dropped. Our fellow passengers averted their eyes. In the reception area, I caught a glimpse of Ricky Lee looking brightly about her. Anyone watching us would be watching Ricky Lee. She was waiting for me, ergo I was still upstairs. The leather-faced policeman was arguing with the woman behind the reception desk. I did not want to leave Ricky Lee there. But

I hunched my shoulders and pushed the chair down a hallway that led in the opposite direction. Time was short.

There were other wheelchairs waiting like supermarket trolleys in the parking lot. John clambered into the car on his hands and knees, eased himself groaning into the passenger seat. He laid his head on the headrest and closed his eyes. I wound the seatback down and threw a rug over him. Then I drove out of the car park and out of town at one-eighth of a mile an hour under the speed limit.

I cruised gently east, keeping my eye on the rearview mirror. We had impersonated FBI personnel. We had resisted arrest, aided and abetted a suspect in evading custody. But police cars were not the main worry. The main worry was T-shirts with fists on them.

The mirror stayed empty. The buildings fell away; the road ran straight as an arrow. The cornlands began to give way to grassy hills. I began to relax. The road curved south to avoid a large expanse of water. There were trees now, and woods. I said, "Do you want another hospital?"

"Hell no," he said.

I made a business stop in Meadville. We bought John a Pittsburgh Steelers cap to cover his bandages. The visible parts of his face were too pale. I was worried about him. There was a pay phone in a gray cement street. With it I called the hospital and asked for X-ray. I told them I was in Canada, and that if John died his heirs would sue. They told me the X-rays showed no fracture. I slammed the phone down, bought a couple of sandwiches at a general store, and climbed back into the car.

John had levered himself into yesterday's clothes and cranked his seatback vertical. Except for the bandages, he looked as normal as he was ever going to look. I twisted the starter. He said, "What we doing?"

"Driving to Portland," I said. "Pick up the car. Want a sandwich?"

He shook his head, winced. "Feels like my brain's loose," he said. We drove northeast and joined the freeway west of Erie. Beyond a flat foreshore dotted with tacky chalets, the westering sun was blazing a tangerine-colored trail across the lake. The car felt secure, inviolable.

John popped the cassette out of the player, fiddled with the radio, found a country station.

There was a flatpicked guitar, a man's voice, high lonesome backing singers.

> I been out of luck.
> I been down so long I feel like the feathers
> On a duck

The chorus repeated. The DJ said, "The late great Rhydian Walters, ladies and gentlemen."

I shoved the Sullivan cassette into the player. I played "Birdman in the Corn" and switched it off. I said, "What do you think?"

"About what?"

"'Birdman in the Corn.'"

He frowned. "It's a song, right?"

"What does it mean?"

He shrugged.

I said, "We have just been to see J. J. Birdman, the corn merchant."

His head snapped around. His mouth was a red hole in his beard.

I said, "Why do you think Rhyd wrote that?"

John said, "I dunno. Jeez." He was silent for five miles. Then he said, "He was right."

"About what?"

"He spoke real high of you. He said you understood things other people didn't understand, which was what made you a real poet, which he never would be."

I was so surprised my ears were ringing. He was talking about Rhyd, who could do anything he wanted to do. I knew about sailing boats and writing poems and the private life of birds. Trivial stuff. Rhyd and Camilla had had their hands on the lever that made the world spin.

John said, "He never told you that?"

I said, "Not in so many words." It had not been the kind of thing Rhyd did tell people. He and Camilla had trusted me with their children and treated me as a friend. But neither of them had been the kind of personalities you could imagine comparing themselves adversely with anyone else. For a moment the sense of loss came back, full power.

"So what's with this song?" said John. "That got something to do with what happened?"

I pulled myself back to the present. I said, "Yes."

"How?"

"We have a government agency that puts a marker on some corn," I said. "The corn is being sent abroad as part of an aid consignment. Rhyd is sending messages back about this consignment. You were out there. Did he ever talk about any of this?"

John thought about it, frowning heavily against the headache. "Maybe. I was telling you when you came over to the boat. Rhyd used to sail with me when charter wasn't so good, and, you know, a diving boat is kind of an expensive thing to keep on the water? So I was doing this stuff. That's why they call me Scotch John."

"What stuff?"

He seemed oddly bashful. He said, "It's real basic. In spring I go up to Rhodes, right? Up in Rhodes, Scotch comes in at fifteen dollars a bottle in bond, Johnny Walker, Chivas, all correct. So I was bringing this stuff down to Port Sudan, trading it with this guy. He was giving me like sixty bucks a bottle? Bring in fifty cases, you're talking serious money. So anyways, this guy would pay me partly in money and partly in dope, right? So we'd have this big bale of bush, all wrapped up in plastic, and we'd take that sucker out at night and we'd heave it overboard, just south of Egyptian territorial waters. So the breeze would float it up over the border, and this police launch would find it."

"Police launch?"

"You learn a lesson," said John. It was dark, now. The trees of New York State flickered green and wet in the headlamps. I could almost see the yellow-brown shore, the brilliant turquoise of the Red Sea. "When you're down that way, you don't trust nobody. But if you got something that will make money, you are best off going to a cop with it, because that way you don't get problems, except maybe from the army."

I said, "Where does Rhyd come into this?"

"Into the dope? Nowhere," he said. He sounded shocked. "Just absolutely stone nowhere. Not directly, anyway. After I'd been doing this a while, looking good, you know, a guy comes up from the south. A cop called Eugene Wollo. Things had gone quieter in Eritrea, things were opening up, he said. Could I find him some whiskey? He was quite a fixer, this guy. He's been working down in Mitsiwa, at the north end of Ethiopia. So I started to work with this guy. Whiskey for dynamite bush. Everything went through Eugene. The dope was a nice little sideline for him; low effort, high margin. That was when Rhyd got interested."

"How?"

"We was sitting in Port Sudan on the boat, drinking a beer. There was a big mother of a grain ship alongside in the commercial dock, break-bulk cargo, because it had to go on these terrible bush trucks they have down there. And there was the Red Cross trucks, and the UNICEF trucks, and they were all loading up and rolling out of the docks, away south, where folks were starving gently to death, and there's a relief operation going down. And in among the international good guys, there is this other bunch of trucks that belong to Wollo. And we see them pallets of bags going on to these trucks. But when they get to the harbor gate, instead of hitting the road south, they are making a right. So Rhyd says, let's go look at these guys. So we call a taxi and the taxi follows one of Eugene's trucks. And where it goes is a ways north of the town, to this big steel shed that also belongs to Wollo. Some of this grain is going out again to the starving guys. But there are all these other guys with little trucks waiting at the shed. And these guys are not into famine relief, because there is every single grain merchant and baker's store in East Africa queued up there, and they are paying Wollo five dollars a bag, I dunno, for this grain that the honest citizens of the Western world have donated." He laughed, winced. "Good business," he said. "Fifty percent of everything that traveled on his trucks went into his pocket. So, anyway, a while after that, last summer, I put the boat on a rock. They have real bad buoyage out there. Abeba got drowned." He fell quiet, watching the headlights skid across the flat surface of a lake. "There was no insurance. So I came back to the States. Rhyd helped me back. He paid me to refit *Halcyon*, made me a gift of that old tug. He was real good to me."

"Why was he so interested in this Wollo?"

"Listen," said John. "I got one aim in life: stay weightless. Rhyd was a heavy dude. He wanted to feed the world as well as play guitar. He wanted Wollo's ass, because Wollo was starving people. Maybe there was more to it than that. I didn't ask."

My eyes felt like coffee saucers. I thought about Rhyd and Camilla, diving on the coral gardens of the Red Sea. Leaving the heavy burdens of their lives behind. Getting weightless.

But there were other mental pictures. There was Rhyd, sitting in a taxi outside a big shed watching trucks loaded with fat sacks of corn trailing white plumes of dust away into the interior. It would have been gritty in the back of the taxi. The dust would have mixed with the sweat at the nape of his neck, turned his ballpoint pen into a little mill wheel, grinding on the paper. Mill wheels within mill wheels. Everyone had something to grind.

I said, "And what about Ras Hamil?"

"Ras who?"

"Ras Hamil. Did Rhyd ever talk about him?"

"Rhyd knew what I was into. He only talked about what he needed me to know."

I thought about the consignment of corn marked with radioactive iodine by the Emergency Resources Bureau. I thought of it bagged up at J. J. Birdman, loaded on to a ship for Port Sudan, glowing invisibly in the hold. Unloaded in the dust and glare of Port Sudan. Taken out to the big shed, owned by Eugene Wollo, proprietor of J. J. Birdman's consignee company.

I said, "And Wollo's company was called Aid Services."

John turned his head slowly. "Like Rhyd said." he said. "You understand things other people don't understand."

I understand a lot. But very little of it made any sense. Wearily, I shoved Rhyd's cassette back into the slot.

22

COUNTRY SONGS ARE SIMPLE OBJECTS, AS POEMS GO. THEY ARE descended from Appalachian mountain tunes, which are descended in their turn from European folk songs brought over by early settlers. Country music is folk music for suburbia, founded on nostalgia for the simple wisdoms of a rural Golden Age that probably never existed.

Rhyd's particular version hinged on a gnomic chorus line or couplet. The material of the verses expanded the theme expressed in the chorus and supplied a narrative thread. I had written an article to this effect for *Acta Poetica*.

But I had never before attempted to use literary criticism to delve into the background of aid fraud and bloody murder.

Catalogue first.

Three tracks on the tape. First, "Birdman in the Corn." Then "Mr. Coffee":

> Come down and drink a beer with Mr. Coffee,
> Let Mr. Coffee take you by the hand.
> Have yourself some fun

CLAWHAMMER

With Mr. Coffee's gun
And die with Mr. Coffee in the sand.

The verses were a portrait of Mr. Coffee, who supplied
money to people who did not need it with one hand while
strangling their children with the other.

"Cash crops," I said.

"Huh?" said John.

For years, Ethiopians had their own coffee, on land that was
right for it. Lately, farmers had been persuaded by traders to
plant coffee on marginal land. Their coffee price had plummeted, the land was exhausted, the farmers starved. It was a
typical Rhyd theme.

No secrets.

The next song was the version of "The Alleluia Tree,"
Rhyd's great triumphal anthem. It was one of Rhyd's many
pickup-truck songs, with resonances of the Theseus and the
Minotaur story. It concerned a woman whose husband ran off
with a floozie. The woman trawled the bars for the adulterer
and found him soaking up remorseful bourbons at a table by
himself. He promised to come home and started back in his car,
with instructions to leave the house's outside light on. Being
drunk, he passed out on the porch without turning the light
on. The wife, seeing the house in darkness, thought he had
deserted her, and drove her pickup truck spang into the trunk
of the Alleluia Tree, killing herself. The tree the next morning
was seen to be bearing, for the first and only time, blood-red
flowers.

This version had the new verse:

When the Book of Life is written
To which this is the key,
The Lord will post it in the library
By the Alleluia Tree.

I played it again. It still sounded like neo-Apocalyptic
gibberish. I said, "Did he ever tell you about an Alleluia Tree?"

211

"Sure," said John. "It was in that village where he was."

I knew about that one. "Nothing else?"

"Should there be?"

It was raining now. I watched the road through the windscreen wipers. I thought about the key to the Book of Life. It was not a particularly Rhyd Walters notion. His style ran more to pickup trucks and whiskey.

"So," said John. "Where we at?"

He sounded as if he expected me to have it all worked out. "There's a J. J. Birdman song," I said. "An anti-cash-crop song. And a Book of Life verse on 'The Alleluia Tree.'"

"So?" said John.

"We are looking for the big dirt on Ras Hamil," I said. "Any lawyer in America will tell you that this is not it."

The tape played on.

The words of "Birdman in the Corn" had Rhyd's usual conversational fluency. But after I had heard the last verse ten times, I found I was frowning.

> So she handed him a number,
> Said, "Quit looking so forlorn.
> I'm off to Quebec, Papa,
> With the birdman in the corn."

The second and third lines sounded wrong. In the second line, the syllables were crammed in like sardines in a tin. He could just as easily have sung "don't look" instead of "quit looking." In the third line, the initial consonants of the last two words tripped the voice, lost fluency.

The initial consonants.

I fumbled in my shirt pocket. I handed John the paper I had scribbled on at Birdman's. I said, "Four four seven two seven QP."

John said, *"What?"*

"Read the paper."

He turned on the inside light. He said, "Four four seven two seven QP. You remembered that?"

I said, "It's in the song. The numbers of letters in the words of the second line. Then the radio phonetic alphabet equivalents for Q and P."

John said, "What's it for?"

"Rhyd was sending Bill information. He would have set it up beforehand with Bill. That's how Bill got the consignment number." The one I had seen in Ricky Lee's notebook.

"But we got it," said John. "And it still ain't the big dirt. You want to think about those other songs?"

I said, "I'm thinking."

But it was one thing to making a puzzle tally with a known fact. It was entirely another starting from scratch.

We drove on in silence. It was getting late. On the tape player, Rhyd sang on. The freeway unrolled, dotted on either side by the blink of houses between the trees. I thought John was asleep.

It must have been an hour before he spoke. He said, "Was Rhyd trying to get information home to bust Aid Services?"

I said, "Can you see Rhyd working for the U.S. government?"

"No way," he said.

That was the first problem. The second was that Rhyd and Camilla had been murdered by Ras Hamil, not Eugene Wollo. So if the murder and the flour sample were related, there must be a connection between Hamil the warlord and Wollo the cop.

Assume there was a connection. Assume Rhyd had found what it was. Assume Rhyd had not been working for any government. Assume he had decided to hand Bill a story. Bill had been on his way to Ethiopia when Ras Hamil had killed Rhyd and Camilla to silence them. But Rhyd had left a sample of flour for Bill and had sent off tapes of coded information when he knew his life was in danger.

And on his way home to collect the information, Bill had been shot by drug smugglers.

Lucky for someone. Perhaps for the someone who employed Gerard and Jackson. In which case, why had Gerard and Jackson left me alive?

My foot was aching on the accelerator. Beyond the white pool of the headlamps, the night was black as tar. I felt naked, floodlit on a great flat plain with no hiding places, nowhere to go but on into the middle of the fear. The word was committed, the way a bomb is committed after it has been dropped. Rhyd and Camilla would have congratulated me.

Speaking as the bomb, I was not so sure congratulations were in order.

We picked up the Mustang from Portland airport and turned in the hire car. We arrived back at Quogue in the late afternoon. The harbor was flat as asphalt, cloaked in haze. Quogue Island was a gray whaleback whose edges receded into a gray blur. John had been asleep most of the way. Daylight made things seem less dangerous. I picked up some mail from Danny, told John to get some sleep. I stumbled into the dory and pulled for *Halcyon*.

I went below, posted a few split logs into the stove and started on the bundle of letters. I began at the top of the pile, worked my way down through the envelopes, looking for the boys' writing. The stove filled the cabin with the smell of hot iron. There were a couple of fan letters forwarded by Pierce, one of them apologizing for not being able to make a cash donation and offering carnal knowledge in lieu. There was a letter from Julia the editor, telling me that my dilatoriness was endangering the success of the entire ducks project. I wondered what Julia would say if she knew exactly how endangered the ducks project was.

The last envelope in the pile was addressed in my own handwriting. I blinked at the fog in my head. If it was in my own writing, what was it doing on my table?

I stopped blinking. My heart turned over in my chest and walloped against my ribs.

It was addressed to Masters Joe and Harry Walters at Pleasant Lake Camp. The names were crossed out. Someone had written in blue pencil "RETURN TO SENDER—NOT KNOWN AT THIS ADDRESS."

I pulled on a pair of shoes and a sweater and pounded up the companionway and into the evening. It took ten minutes to row across to the telephone. The fog was bad. A pair of eider ducks were floating nearly invisible in the black reflections under the quay pilings. They took off as I approached, a pair of winged bottles thrashing back to their simple world: eat, breed, don't get dead. I crammed money into Danny's pay phone.

The telephone rang long and hard at the end of a line that hissed like a serpent. The echoes of its bell would be crashing from the varnished surfaces of the high, bare rooms.

The ringing stopped. There was a silence, in which I could hear the blood whining in my ears. A woman's voice said, "Who's that?"

"George Devis," I said.

"Oh." The word fell like a brick in the silence.

I said, as calmly as I could, "I've been trying to get in touch with the boys."

She said, "We told you. They're in camp."

I breathed deeply. I said, "No, they are not."

She said sharply, "How do you know?"

"I wrote to the address you gave me. The camp sent the letter back."

"Oh," she said, without any emotion I could detect.

The blood was roaring in my ears. *Don't blow it,* I told myself. I said, "Where are they?"

She said, "You can't know."

I said, "I have a right to know."

She put the telephone down.

I dialed again with a hand that shook. The telephone rang for twelve minutes by my watch. I walked out, managed a wave at Danny, climbed into the car. I began to drive north.

I drove like hell. Camilla and Rhyd were dead. Joe and Harry were alive, and too young to look after themselves.

Out on the highway, my pulse slowed to a hard, steady thump. The lights of other cars were irregular globes of haze. I was on my own, like the boys. I was going to take them away from that hellhole and set them free.

Nothing else mattered.

23

I TURNED DOWN THE TRACK INTO BETHEL AT ELEVEN O'CLOCK. THE headlights glinted faintly off the ponds. There were no lights in the house, only a dim yellow square slipping behind the branches of the trees from the general direction of the gable end of the barn. Chuck was at home. My hands became damp on the wheel. He was probably oiling his guns.

I drove into the yard, climbed out of the car and turned off the lights. The darkness was complete. Chuck's window was in the gable end of the barn, facing out of the yard. The sea crunched on the shore, and the wind that whispers in pines whispered in the pines. A dog was barking in a shed somewhere. A thread of country music wound through the breeze. There was Rhyd's solid flat-picked guitar, the lazy howdy-doody voice. A commercial recording: "Children, Don't Play with Daddy's Glass Eye, He Needs It to Look for Work." There was a banjo track on it. I did not remember a banjo track on the original. I walked up the porch steps and hauled on the pull of the bell. A yellow square of window shone above. Feet stumped on to a wooden floor, clattered down stairs. A voice the other side of the door said, "Who's that?"

Sarah's voice.

"George Devis."

She paused. She said, "Go 'way."

I said, "I'm not going away until you tell me what you've done with the boys."

"No."

The anger was bubbling like volcanic mud. I said, "We are joint guardians. If you do not open up I will be back here in four hours with my lawyer."

She said, "Are you alone?"

The dog was barking harder. I would not be alone long. Chuck would be keeping me company. Him and his gun and his faulty ten-year-old's memory. I said, "Yes."

There was a rattle of bolts and chains. The door opened. Light streamed into the fog, dazzling me. I walked in.

She was wearing a green-gray wool dressing gown and plaid bedroom slippers. Her hair hung loose on her shoulders. Her face looked gray and strained, the eyes open a quarter of an inch too wide, the mouth lipless, stretched downward at the corners. She said, "Why are you pursuing us like this?"

I said, "I'm pursuing Joe and Harry. I want to know where they are."

She said, "It's none of your business."

I said, "I am their co-guardian."

She held my eye. Her mouth was shut, pale as an old scar. She knew I was right. She tried a smile. It was not convincing. "They're at camp," she said.

I breathed deeply. Be logical. Do not let yourself think that the boys are the last of your family, the last link with Camilla. I said, "That's what you told me last time."

The smile became ghastly. "Change of . . . plan," she said. "We decided on another."

I said, "You lied to me."

She said, "You wouldn't have understood."

I hung on tight. I said, "How do you know?"

She lifted her hands, let them fall again. "You can't," she said. "You're not . . ." Her voice trailed away.

"One of the Elect."

She raised her eyes. There was a hint of warmth in the clamminess, but only a small one. "Rhydian did speak good of you, one time," she said. "But you can't understand what this means to us folks."

I said, "I thought Rhyd was lost to you."

She said, "Rhydian was a grown man. We are taught to teach our children the straight and narrow path."

I thought of the names in new ink in the family Bible. My heart was thudding in my chest. Calm, I told myself. I said, as mildly as I could, "Under the terms of the will, we have joint responsibility. Unless you abide by those terms, you are not honoring your side of the agreement. In which case, a court could investigate your circumstances. You could end up with no control over the boys at all."

She stared at me with her too-wide eyes. The spark of warmth had vanished.

"Also," I said, "I don't know if this matters to you, but the boys have had a tough enough time as it is without being squabbled over."

She said, quickly, "There are more important things than earthly desires."

I said, "Maybe I did not make myself clear. I want to talk to the people who are looking after the boys. Now."

She was wringing her hands. "Well," she said. "Maybe I could call in the morning—"

I said, "If I do not get to talk to the boys, my lawyers will be here in the morning."

She said, in a dead voice, "I cannot reasonably refuse."

My stomach turned over. She was quoting from the will. In the bottom of my mind had been the hope that she was doing what she was doing out of ignorance and half-bakedness. From now on, it was going to be the letter of the law.

On her side, anyway.

Feet thundered on the porch steps. The brass fender in front of the black iron stove rattled. Chuck came in.

He had the usual equipment. There was the mouth, ajar,

with the bead of slobber forming at the sump of the lower lip. There was the Machias Freezer baseball cap, pulled down far enough to jug the ears. There was his best friend the rifle. I ignored the drool and the headgear and concentrated on the rifle. His thick finger lay alongside the trigger guard. Ready for anything.

Sarah looked up, telephone in hand. She said, "Not in the house, Chuckie," in the soft voice she kept for him.

Chuck scowled. He said, "What's he want?" with his big pauses between words, as if there were teeth missing from the cogs in his mind.

"Visiting," said Sarah, with a desperate attempt at a smile. "Hello," she said to the telephone. "Is that Greenbank?" Her eyes swiveled at me. I grinned at Chuck, and said, "Actually, I came to see the boys."

Chuck nodded blankly. "They ain't here," he said.

"Sure," I said. "They give you a hard time?"

"They went where they wasn't allowed to go," he said. "My barn."

"So they pissed you off, right?"

"Yeah." Chuck nodded. "I keep my stamps up there. My collection. It don't need to be all messed up."

"No," I said.

"They was climbing everywheres," said Chuck. "Up my barn. Everywheres around. Until they went to camp. Nosy kids."

I shoved my hands in my pockets, clenched the fists to stop myself wrapping his rifle around his neck.

Sarah looked up from the telephone. She said, "You want to talk to them?"

That surprised me. "Of course," I said.

"They'll go fetch them."

There was a silence. Chuck had laid the rifle on a couple of pegs on the wall. He was humming a song. I relaxed a little.

"Okay," said Sarah. She had herself under control now. She was smiling, a bright, air-hostessy smile. It looked ridiculous. She gave me the telephone.

I said, "Who's there?"

A voice said, "Me." Even through the hiss of the Bethel Bay line it was undoubtedly Joe. I felt a sudden surge of affection and relief. I said, "Are you all right? And Harry?"

"Yes," he said. He did not elaborate, which was not like him.

I said, "Where are you?"

"Nice place," he said. "It's got every amenity."

I said, "Really?"

This was a family joke. The last place I had heard him describe as having every amenity was a new slaughterhouse they were building on the Pulteney Industrial Estate. He was using the double-talk because there was someone else in the room.

Joe said, "How are you?"

I told him I was a TV star, and other half-truths. I wanted to find out how he was. I said, "Have you been sailing?"

"Canoeing," he said.

River or lake. "And a bit of religious instruction?"

"Just a bit," he said. "Very edifying." Sarcasm had always been his middle name. "I must go. Harry wants a word."

Harry was more direct. He said, "Come and get us out of here. Please." He was hanging on to himself, just. He had had practice, these last few months.

I said, "We're working on it," before they could yank the receiver out of his hand.

There was a scuffle going on at the far end. "Cool," he said, diminuendo. The telephone turned slippery in my hand. I found I was shouting his name.

The man's voice said, "Nice talking to you, sir."

The line went dead.

"See?" said Sarah. "They're fine."

It was slipping away from me. I said, "No, they bloody well are not fine. I want them out of that place, wherever it is. Within twenty-four hours."

She said, "You can bring your lawyers, but I am advised that you will not prevail."

"Elder Hornbeck said," said Chuck.

She was staring at me with her cold gray eyes. I recognized the finality in the set of her jaw. Rhyd had held his jaw like that, except with him it had signified resolution, not pigheadedness.

Chuck walked into the corner with his clumsy pneumatic-man waddle, picked up the gun and looked as if he felt better. He might find words complicated, but he had an excellent understanding of atmospheres. We were across the Rubicon now. I took a deep breath. I said, "Well, then. When can I see the boys?"

She relaxed. I had seen reason. She said, "End of basic training. I'll call you. There's no way of telling."

"Sure," I said, looking at Chuck, who was looking at me. I grinned at them both. The grin was insincere, but the baring of teeth was not. There were two thoughts in my mind, one hard to grasp, the other not. The hard one was why Rhydian should have thought for one second that this woman was a sensible co-guardian for his children.

The easy one was that if Sarah believed I was going to waive visiting rights till the end of basic training, she would be off her guard.

And she would be in for a shock.

24

IN RED HILL, A LIGHT WAS BURNING IN THE PORCH OF THE GENERAL store, illuminating a petrol pump and the flaking green paint of the building's front. The diner was full of steam and dirty chrome. Mrs. Rider was still flowing over the rim of her ski pants, still wearing her giant sneakers. On the TV, a glossy woman was bellowing at a man in a silver toupee. The volume dial was turned up to nine. A couple of men in check shirts were watching, backs to the bar.

"Hi there," bellowed Mrs. Rider with enthusiasm. "How you doin'?"

I could hardly hear her over the TV. She pressed a remote control. The volume dropped. "Gen'l'men bin working in the sawmill. Saw noise gits their ears."

I ordered a beer. I said, "Have you ever heard of a place around here called Greenbank?"

She shook her head, wobbling some chins.

It was not amazing. The Brethren had the whole U.S.A. to site their boot camp in.

"Seen Joe and Harry," she said.

"When was that?" I said.

"They come in here to stock up," she said. "Maybe a week ago. That little guy, Harry, right? He said he was going on a trip, he needed big supplies. I was telling him, way he was going, I wondered would his teeth hold out. He said he guessed where he was going they'd pull all his teeth out anyway." She eased the elastic of her ski pants from her third to her fourth roll of stomach. "Real funny little guy," she said.

I said, "He didn't say where he was going?"

"Yeah," she said. "Bangor. Someplace close to Bangor."

So there we were. Nice, unimaginative Brethren. Greenbank, close by Bangor. A hundred miles away, if that. Near a river or lake.

She shook her head. "I'd be glad they was out of there," she said. "Bethel, I mean. That Chuck. He gives me the shivers. I mean, poor guy and all, but ugh." She shivered like an earthquake. The door opened. Her curranty eyes were looking past me. "Greenbank," she said, ruminatively.

"Greenbank where?" said a voice.

I turned around. Of course, it was Ricky Lee.

She was wearing jeans and a checked shirt. She came over and pulled out a bar stool and sat down on it, back to the bar, leaning it back on two legs, propping her elbows on the bar counter. She hooked the heels of her cowboy boots in the stretcher and dropped her chin on her chest, acting out a minor crucifixion. Then she grinned at me. She looked tired, but pleased. She said, "You look the way I feel."

I smiled back at her. I did not feel like smiling at anyone, but it was hard not to smile at her. I had a moment of what felt like telepathic communication. I was not alone, and she was not alone, and we were both pleased about it, and we knew it. I ordered her a beer. She seemed pleased about that, too.

I said, "Is this an accident?"

She said, wearily, "Finding people is my job. I'm good at it." The beer arrived, no glass. She took a swig out of the bottle. "Oof," she said. The skin under her eyes was dark, and there were razor-thin lines bracketing the corners of her mouth. "It's a long way from Cleveland."

"What happened?"

She smiled, ironically. "I got arrested."

"Is that all?"

Her eyebrows went up. "All?" she said. "Accessory after the fact of aiding and abetting resisting arrest. Who pays the lawyers?"

"Me?"

She put her hand on my hand. It seemed the natural place for it. "I'll stick the *Echo*," she said.

"I'm sorry."

She said, "I walked into it with my eyes open." Her mouth turned down at the corners. "And there were only cops involved."

"Only."

"No prizefighters. Just ten hours in the interview room, and my immortal soul in danger." She drank again.

I said, "How did you find me?"

She yawned. She said, "Scotch John said he guessed you might have left for Bethel Bay. It will not have escaped your attention that there is only one road to Bethel Bay, with not a hell of a lot of candy-apple-red Mustangs on it."

"Smart," I said.

She said, "You have to be smart if you want a staff job on the *Echo*." She looked at me straight and hard. Her eyes were green as a cat's. "Besides, there aren't too many nice guys in my life right now."

The people on the television had stopped talking. The words echoed around the room. The sawmill workers kept their eyes on the screen, waiting for the lips to start moving again.

She dropped her eyes, took a sip of her beer. I took a sip of mine. The something between us was moving out from cover into open ground.

She said, "So what about Greenbank?"

I said, "The boys are there."

She said, "Oh." She looked into her glass. The subject had changed. Her mouth was turned down at the corners. She said, "What do you know about this place?"

I said, "It's a boot camp for Christ's Brethren."

"That's right."

I said, "How do you know?"

She did not look up. She said, "I used to be there."

The sawmill men bellowed goodnights at Mrs. Rider. Mrs. Rider said, "It's okay, I ain't closing," and twinkled like a Christmas pudding.

I said, "Why?"

She said, "My mom sent me there."

I waited.

She said, "My daddy died. My mom met this guy. He was one of the Brethren, right? Greenbank's the place they send you to get anointed."

"Anointed?"

"The Brethren," she said. "They're the Lord's Anointed. They don't like to admit that anyone outside themselves actually exists. But they can see that in, like, special circumstances, people want to keep their kids, so they have to bend the kids around."

"Bend them around." I could hear Joe and Harry's voices on the telephone; the relief at hearing a voice from outside. "Are you sure?"

She said, "This is not a fun place." She drank more beer. Her face was stony and exhausted. For the first time since I had known her, it was without humor. "Why do you think I am on this story?"

I watched her. Her eyes were angry and haunted-looking. I said, "I think you'd better tell me."

She smiled. It was a hard, twisted smile, not like her real one. She said, "It's not easy to talk about the Brethren."

I thought of Rhyd, silent all those years, willing his sons into captivity. I said, "I've noticed."

She said, "There was a party. It was a kind of music party. Hud Krantz was there. He used to be Rhyd's manager. Actually, that was why I was there too. I wanted to meet Hud, give him a tape of some songs I'd written. I kind of admired Rhyd. I mean I didn't know him, but he'd made it away from the

Brethren, and I'd known his sister and all that. And I guess I thought this tape was like a memorial for Maria. Anyway, at this party Hud was busy, like those kind of guys are at parties. Actually, he was talking to Bill. And he introduced me to Bill and, like, sidled away to network a little. So that left Bill and me. I'd met Bill before, but he didn't remember me, I guess. We were talking about Rhyd. And Bill said he knew Rhyd, so I said I had known Maria. So then we started talking about the Brethren and what it was like to get away from them. Bill had a theory that it was like losing your family, that it either killed you or made you stronger than you would have been, but, like, scarred."

I thought about losing families. I wondered which way I was heading.

"So anyway. I told him I had been to journalism school and he asked me to work with him. So of course I did, because Bill was really a good reporter, famous."

I said, "How did the story involve the Brethren?"

She said, "I told you, Bill was gabby like a clam. But he had this method. He said that if you were writing a big story, you needed not just facts in depth; you needed characters, too, to make your readers understand how the facts fitted in with the lives. So he had to get into the Brethren question." She shrugged. "So that made it a wonderful job for me. A rung on the ladder, and a labor of love." She looked at me sideways from the slanted eyes. "Not that kind of love," she said. "Strictly professional. Bill used those parts of me he needed. My dialing finger, my notebook. That's all."

I was relieved. This is ridiculous, I thought. What are you relieved about?

She said, "So you want to go to Greenbank?"

I said, "How about tomorrow morning?"

She said, "It may not be as easy as that."

I tried a smile. It felt stiff and unnatural. I said, "We'll manage. You did."

She said, "It was different then. I just ran away."

"Just like that?"

She said, "I'd been there a year. They have these deacons, like camp guards. There are a lot of kids there. You have Education and Doctrine. You do anything they don't like, they beat up on you. If someone tells you black's white, and beats up on you when you argue, you pretty soon start to agree. It's like . . . being deformed suddenly, like in a dream. It's a terrible idea. The most terrible thing about it is that you get used to it. So after you've agreed for a while, you begin to believe it. Specially when you're a little kid."

I was cold as ice. I said, "What happened?"

"I found a *Cosmopolitan* in the principal's garbage."

"*Cosmopolitan?*"

"The problem page. It was all about sex. They didn't talk about sex at Greenbank. I was thirteen. I was thinking about it a whole lot. It made me realize the world outside added up with the way I was feeling and the world inside didn't. So outside was sane and inside was crazy, which was the other way around from what they were telling us inside. So I went over the fence. That was a long time ago. They've got razor wire on it now. You won't get them out without dynamite."

The way I was feeling, dynamite sounded fine. Dynamite and maybe a lawyer.

"And . . ." she said. She met my eyes again, tentatively.

"Yes?"

"I should remind you that according to your schedule you have a lecture tomorrow evening. In Lexington, Massachusetts."

I nodded. The George Devis who gave lectures and raised funds seemed as remote as Christopher Columbus. We walked out into the Maine night.

I followed the little red eyes of Ricky Lee's rear lights until she pulled into the yard of a motel. We took adjoining cabins. Next morning, I woke up to a tapping on my door. It was Ricky Lee, with two paper cups of coffee. She handed me one, and sat on the bed. She said, "What are you going to do?"

I said, "Find a lawyer. Go and see the boys."

"Do you have a lawyer?"

"No."

"There was the guy I had. George Caziris. He has an office in Boston. He . . . sprung me. Or anyway he made it so I didn't have to go back."

"How long ago?"

"Ten years. He's still around. He's a good friend."

I said, "What's his number?"

She wrote it on a piece of paper. I carried it along to the pay phone in the hall.

It was barely eight, but George Caziris was already at work. He had a voice like the Mustang's idle. I explained that my two nephews were at Greenbank. He said, "How did you get my number?"

"Ricky Lee Klaasen."

He made a noise that could have been a laugh. "Alumni week," he said. "She tell you I got her out of there? Well, she got herself out of there, and I kept her out."

"She told me."

"So," he said. "You're their uncle, huh?"

I explained that I was also their co-guardian.

"With whom?"

I explained about Sarah Ebden.

"And she has them for this portion of the year, right? Under the terms of a will? You got it with you?"

I quoted it to him.

"You have a problem," he said. "Unless you can show your co-guardian is insane or delinquent, you don't have a chance. And whatever you or I may think, being of the Brethren is not prima facie evidence of either. Sure, we can go into this if you have time. Statements from witnesses. Psychiatrists' reports." He coughed. I heard the fizz of a lighter, the hiss as he inhaled. "But if you're getting them back anyway, it's kind of long drawn out. You might as well wait, right?"

He had a point. But Joe and Harry were in there, being brainwashed. I said, "What if I took them away?"

Caziris said, "This would be very illegal." He sighed, "Would I be right in thinking you're going to do it anyway?"

I did not answer.

He said, "It would certainly make things . . . more difficult."
He exhaled noisily.

"Thank you," I said.

"Anything for Ricky Lee," he said. "Oh, by the way."

"Yes."

"Good luck."

25

*G*REENBANK WAS VISIBLE FROM TWO MILES AWAY. IT WAS A LARGE wooden edifice, set aggressively on top of a low, rocky hill in a landscape of other low hills. Blackish waves of pines rolled up to its walls. We drove along a single-track road until our way was blocked by an eight-foot gate in a chainlink fence topped with a coil of razor wire. Ricky Lee sat white and pale in the passenger seat. There was a telephone on the right-hand gatepost. I climbed out of the car, picked it up. My mouth felt dry as cotton wool. A voice asked me who I was. I gave my name and told it I had come to visit Joe and Harry Walters.

"Joseph and Henry are particularly engaged right now," said the voice.

I said, "I've come a long way."

The voice said it was sorry.

I said, "For the children's sake, I'd like to keep this discreet. Otherwise I'll be back, and I'll be bringing some TV cameras and some reporters and a lawyer called George Caziris."

The voice put me on hold for five minutes. Just as I thought I had been abandoned, it came back on the line. "I'm so sorry," it said. "There was a mistake. Won't you come right on up?"

An automatic latch buzzed. The gate swung open. I drove through. "Christ, this place," said Ricky Lee. She was looking around her, chewing her thumbnail.

Normally, when you go back to someone's childhood stamping ground, they reminisce. But Ricky Lee tucked her head into her shoulders, blank-faced and miserable, as the road wound up through the dappled shade of the trees.

A lake opened out on the right. Its water was dirty brown. Canoes were pulled up on the banks. A group of children were walking across a patch of grass, hands folded in front of them, eyes lowered.

" 'A modest gaze, and hands in view, undoes what the Devil wills you do,' " said Ricky Lee, with sourness. "No swimming, either. You can get impure thoughts from swimming. Specially when you're thirteen."

The road ran away from the lake up to the front of the building. It was a single block, four stories high and perhaps 150 feet across the front. Its clapboard walls were white. The paint was flaking, as if the Brethren had saved their housekeeping budget for the razor wire. It was a slab-sided, unforgiving lump of a building, with high sash windows that gave it an air of idiotic surprise.

A door opened in the center of the front wall; a white door, with no frame or porch or step. It looked as bald and sinister as an eye with no brows or lashes. A man appeared.

He stood in the door and waited. He had little blue eyes. His whole face ran outward to a nose with an end like a pair of tiny buttocks and a wet little mouth full of backward-sloping teeth. He was pink and pear-shaped, wearing a white shirt, no tie, buttoned at the collar and pushed into a pair of dark gray Terylene trousers. On his feet were well-polished black shoes.

Ricky Lee gripped my arm. She said, "It's the Pig." Her lips looked thin and whitish. "Watch him. He's clever."

We got out. The day was sticky hot, with a smell of pines. I was telling myself: Play this by the book. Collect your evidence. Bide your time. Keep it legal.

The man in the doorway said, "Welcome to Greenbank. I am

Elder Hornbeck." His eyes were flat as coins. He did not offer his hand. If he had, I guessed it would have been cold and wet. The eyes moved away from me on to Ricky Lee. He bared the inward-sloping teeth. He said, "We already met."

"That's right," said Ricky Lee, with a toughness I did not recognize.

" 'I say unto you, that likewise joy shall be in heaven over one sinner that repenteth, more than over ninety and nine just persons, which need no repentance.' "

"Tell the fatted calf he can start making long-range plans," said Ricky Lee. "The person who wants to talk with you is Mr. Devis here."

"We already talked," I said. "On the telephone."

"Of course," he said. "Follow me."

We followed his gray flannel bottom through the door. I felt a hand in mine. It was firm, but cold. Ricky Lee was reliving her childhood, and not having a lot of fun.

Despite the heat of the day, there was a distinct chill inside the building. The smell of pines gave way to the smell of disinfectant. The ceilings were high, the floors bare brown boards. In a corner a line of children were on their knees with big rag buffers, polishing. A small black-iron box stove stood in the middle of the room, supporting a black-iron stovepipe that ran in midair to the wall. I said, "It must be cold in the winter."

The Pig said, "Cold is a *material disability,*" as if he did not suffer from it. The children doing the polishing did not raise their eyes as we passed.

The Pig led us through a succession of high-doored chambers into a big, bare room with a single table in the center of the floor. There were chairs on three sides of the table: one at the end, and a single chair facing two side by side. On the side-by-side chairs sat Joe and Harry. They had prison haircuts and they looked pale.

When they saw me they got up and ran toward me, their sneakers thundering on the bare maple boards. I caught them one under each arm.

"Thank you," said the Pig in a voice like a small whip.

They pulled away from me, became rigid. The grins came off their faces as if someone had flicked a switch.

"Chairs," said the Pig.

They sat down.

"Have a seat," said the Pig. He was smiling; a small, seraphic smile I longed to knock off his fat pink face. He sat down at the head of the table and indicated the chair facing the boys.

I said to Joe, "Joe, this is Ricky Lee. Could you fetch her a chair, please?"

Joe blinked, as if he was waking up. He said, "Oh. Sorry. Of course," and smiled at Ricky Lee, his old smile. The set expression left Ricky Lee's face. She smiled back.

The Pig said, "Sit down, Joseph."

Joe's eyes flicked between us. The look on his face turned to one of agony. I said, "All right, then." I went into the next room and fetched the chair myself. Then I said to the Pig, "I'd like to talk to the boys in private."

The Pig said, "You are in private, sir. Say what you have to say."

"Fine," I said. "How's it going, boys?"

"Great," said Joe, in a voice dead as ditchwater.

"Terrific," said Harry, in a voice if anything deader.

Something had changed around their eyes. When we had come in, they had been dull and flat. Now they were animated by something that looked suspiciously like hope.

"They just love it here," said the Pig.

"We just love it here," said the boys tonelessly. The gleam in the eyes was definite. I looked nervously at the Pig. He seemed to be immune to irony. Joe said, "There is a great big lake." I had seen the lake. It was not a great big lake. "There are canoes."

Harry was warming up. He said, in a voice from beyond the tomb, "The canoes are a groove."

"I have to tell you," said the Pig, "that Joseph and Henry are having a real good time with our outdoor activity program. Huh, guys?"

CLAWHAMMER

"Sure," said Joe.

"Sure," said Harry.

"Entering into the faith of their fathers is like passing through a door into a better world."

I said, "They only had one father. This wasn't his faith."

The boys were both looking at the Pig now. Their faces were blank, but there was hatred in their eyes. *Don't you dare talk about my father,* they were thinking.

The Pig said, "You certainly have a lovely sense of humor, Mr. Devis. Here, we have our eyes fixed on the windows on to the Infinite that are the souls of the Chosen. And I know that our sister Sarah Walters Ebden has her eyes so fixed, in sending these her children in law to be educated in the faith of their . . . er, their spiritual heritage." He paused, pressing his plump palms together as if in prayer. "And we have heard from their own lips that they are pleased with what hath been shewn unto them."

A cold wind seemed suddenly to be blowing on to the base of my skull. Under the terms of the will, if the boys said they wanted to stay in America, they would stay.

"Out of the mouths of babes and sucklings," said the Pig. "Their father strayed from the faith of his fathers. But in his last testament, on the threshold of the next world, he gave his sons the choice. It seems to us that they are choosing, and choosing wisely, to return to the straight way."

I said, "Wait a minute."

"We hear their words. We cannot read the thoughts of their hearts."

Harry said, "They hit you if you tell the truth."

The Pig's cold eyes swung at him. Joe moved in front of his brother. He said, "It's true."

I found I was halfway out of my chair, heading in the general direction of the Pig, and that my fingers were clawed in the strangling position. There was something on my shoulder, digging in. It was Ricky Lee's hand. The boys were looking at me the way drowning people look at life rafts. I sat down again.

"I must make one thing perfectly clear," I said. "If you touch these boys, my lawyer will be issuing writs for common assault. I am at present their co-guardian. I shall be exercising my rights of scrutiny, always assuming it is not possible to extract them from your care and control, such as it is."

The Pig smiled a seraphic smile, and bowed. "It is indeed hard for ye who are Outside to understand the nature of our work."

I said, "It seems pretty straightforward to me. You can expect a visit from my lawyers, as soon as I can arrange it."

"I shall look forward to it," he said.

Ricky Lee's hand pressed mine under the table. *Watch him.*

"One more thing," I said. "This lady is an employee of the Boston *Echo.* A reporter. She has a strong personal and professional interest in stories about the Brethren that concern physical abuse and false imprisonment."

His smile began cracking at the edges. I stood up. "C'mon, boys," I said. "Let's go for a walk. I presume Elder Hornbeck has no objection."

We left the room, all four of us. Harry said, *"Brilliant.* You're a *genius.* Are you really a reporter?"

Joe said, "You want to watch out for that bastard."

"Language."

"He is, though."

We went to the car. I had bought a couple of large bags of supplies, which I distributed. I said, "We've got to go. I'll be back."

Joe nodded. He would not meet my eye. Harry turned away. His excitement had evaporated. He was crying. But he did not complain. He had learned from the events of the past five months that there was no point in complaining, because evil once done stayed done.

I took a deep breath. I was thinking not about Rhyd and his will, but about Camilla. I was thinking about doing the thing you had to do, not the thing you ought to do. There are moments when you live a life according to what the lawyers have advised you to do. There are other moments when you have to throw plans out of the window, even if throwing them is going to make things more difficult for George Caziris.

I turned to Ricky Lee. She was chalk-white behind the freckles. Her eyes looked glassy with tears, as if she was remembering things she had kept down till now.

I said, "How many bedrooms does your house have?"

"Two." She stared at me. She said, "Do it."

I said to the boys, "Get into the car."

Joe looked at the Pig, who was standing in the doorway. Then he looked at me. His face was pale and worried. If there had been a doubt in my mind that I was doing the right thing, it vanished. Anywhere that could frighten Joe this badly was a place he needed to be a long way away from.

He climbed in.

The Pig was ten yards behind us. His mouth was a black circle in his pink face. He said, "Hey?"

I said, "What are you going to do about it?" My ears were singing with rage.

"You are kidnapping these children out of my care and control," he said. His voice had gone tight and piercing. "The gates are locked. I'm calling the police. You are operating outside your legal rights." There were pale children's faces at the windows. He went in. I heard the click of a telephone receiver. Three men came out of the front door. They were big men. They might have been physical fitness instructors or park rangers. They were wearing white nylon shirts buttoned up at the collar, black shoes, and calm Chosen-of-God expressions on their big corn-fed faces.

"Deacons," said Ricky Lee. "Look out."

I climbed into the driver's seat and started the car. The Chosen lumbered into the drive to block the exit. I stamped on the accelerator. Engine howling, the Mustang shot toward them.

Two of them jumped. The third was not quick enough. The wing caught him on the upper leg. He fell across the bonnet, bounced off the windscreen and rolled into a rhododendron bush. In the rearview mirror I could see the other deacons bending over him. I began to feel sick.

"Got Godzilla!" Harry was yelling. "Brilliant!"

Joe was looking out of the back windscreen. "He can stand," he said with regret. He brightened. "But he can't walk."

Ricky Lee was hanging on to my right arm, painfully tight. I flung the Mustang at the curves of the road, spewing gravel into the undergrowth. The lake shot by on the left.

Quietly, Ricky Lee said, "How are you going to get out of the gate?"

I had been thinking about that.

"Free!" Harry was singing. "Free! Hee! Hee! Hee!"

The Mustang slithered around the last corner to the gate. Same old gate, eight feet high, steel and chainlink topped with razor wire, with a remote-operated bolt. A concentration camp gate.

Of course, the gate was shut.

Joe's face was white and frightened. Ricky Lee said, "They'll send the deacons."

Even Harry began to look scared.

I banged on the brakes. The inside of my mouth felt like biscuit-fired clay. I shoved the door open, climbed out.

The telephone was on the left-hand post. There was a gap in the wire so it could be used by people on the way out as well as the way in. I could hear the burble of the Mustang's exhaust, the squeal of a yellow-bellied sapsucker, the rustle of the wind in a clump of maples. The silence of the great outdoors.

For the next two minutes.

I picked up the telephone. The faces in the Mustang were white, screwed around to look for the pursuit.

The Pig's voice in the ear piece said. "Who's that?"

"Piscataquis County Sheriff's Department," I said in the best approximation I could make to a Maine accent. "We had a call, just passing. You folks got a little trouble?"

"Thank goodness," said the voice, slippery as butter. "Come right in. Watch for a red Mustang. The driver is armed and dangerous."

CLAWHAMMER

The gate buzzed. I shoved it. It opened. I jumped into the driver's seat, stamped on the throttle. The fence receded in the rearview mirror.

"Ho, ho, ho," said Harry.

"Shut up," I said. My stomach was hollow, and I was not feeling happy. We were on a single-track oiled dirt road. There would be deacons behind us. There would be police ahead of us. I was supposed to be armed and dangerous, which meant the police might shoot first. There would be charges of assault, kidnapping, contempt of court, reckless driving, and impersonating a police officer.

I said, "Where's the first turnoff?"

"Five miles," said Ricky Lee.

The road ran on between stands of pine. There was an opening on the right: a logging road. I pulled the wheel over. Underbrush scraped the bottom of the car. I pulled in behind a clump of wild raspberries and said, "Get into the wood." They scattered among the tall brown trunks. I went back to the road in the thick green smell of crushed vegetation, brushed the stalks upright. Mosquitoes whined at me. The road had been recently oiled. No tire tracks showed, and there was no dust. Over the rustle of the wood came an undulating wail. I lay down in the bushes below the slope up to the road. A sea-green police car roared past, blue light flaring. The men inside had Roman-coin profiles and moustaches. They did not even glance sideways. I ran back to the car.

It took five minutes to get on to the main road and another forty to get back to Bangor. We transferred to Ricky Lee's car, put the Mustang into a closed parking lot, shoved a couple of hamburgers into the boys, and moved onto the freeway. It was lunchtime. It felt like four o'clock in the morning.

"Ah," said Harry, peeling a Hershey bar with a courtier's elegance. "Luxury."

Ricky Lee leaned across. Her lips were soft on my cheek. She said, "You did great." She hesitated. "Thank you." She was talking for herself, as well as the boys. Her hand stayed on mine. It was warm now.

"Sex rears its ugly head," said Harry.

"Nah," said Joe. "She's not too bad."

I turned around and told them to mind their manners. Ricky Lee was staring straight ahead. She was grinning.

I took her hand and held it. It came to me that I liked Ricky Lee a lot.

That afternoon, we took it in turns to drive the two-hundred-odd miles to her house in Concord. In her tile-and-timber bathroom I shaved off two days' stubble and applied a tie someone had left in her wardrobe to a shirt I had bought that morning in downtown Bangor. Then I went downstairs, called Rooney's in Quogue and asked for Scotch John.

"He's right here," said Danny.

Scotch John said, "Who's that?" His voice sounded slurred.

I said, "You shouldn't be drinking with a concussion."

He said, "Self-medication."

I said, "I have been making myself unpopular in the state of Maine."

"Yeah," he said. "Cops was down here. Rowed all the way out to tell me you was wanted."

"Did they say what the charge was?"

"Assault," said John. "Kidnap."

"Bloody hell," I said.

"Cop said he had to ask you some questions, but he didn't know whether it was a criminal kidnap or a, like, custody dispute. He said they couldn't hang nothing on you."

"Talkative guy," I said.

"I sell him his weed," said John. "This Pierce guy called. Left a number with Danny." He read it out over the telephone. "He said call soon. You okay out there with no bodyguard?"

"I'll keep moving," I said. I gave him Ricky Lee's telephone number. Then I said goodnight to Ricky Lee and the boys, who were watching television, and found Lexington on a map of Greater Boston. It seemed reasonable to assume that Jackson and Gerard considered me successfully warned. The memory of the warning brought me out in a cold sweat. I would be crazy not to be warned.

Perhaps crazy was what I was.

I called Pierce, who asked me to come to his house for a drink before the lecture. I sallied forth on to Highway 2 and into the grown-up world.

The Rapaports lived in the top half of a very big house in a leafy street behind Harvard University. There was a raw-brick stairwell and an oak door that would have been at home in the Cotswolds. Shelagh Rapaport let me in. She had a small tanned face and a big white smile. Tonight her hair was in a dark ponytail. She said, "George!" as if we had known each other all our lives, not just at a quick dinner a week ago. She squeezed my hand. She was wearing a mannish charcoal-gray suit, made out of something that looked like silk, with a necklace that was either made of small lumps of red glass or big rubies.

I followed her across a half-acre floor of polished boards, on which floated an archipelago of oriental rugs. The paintings on the walls were huge. Two of them might have been by Mark Rothko. Under the Rothkos was a square of Danish-looking sofas.

Shelagh brought me a glass of whiskey. She said, "Pierce is on his way." I nodded, and smiled. The Rothkos radiated a quiet gloom over the sofas. Shelagh and I talked about Senator Corin Johanssen, whose wife was sponsoring tonight's lecture.

Pierce came out of an arch fringed with a frieze of scrap-iron trees. "Welcome to Guggenheim North," he said.

Shelagh smiled. "He hates the art," she said.

Pierce said, "You learn to live with it, I guess." He looked as tanned and healthy as his wife. "So how's it been going?"

I told him it had been going fine. He poured himself a good big jolt of the Macallan. He said, "So what did you find?"

I said, "I've tracked the consignment of corn Bill Marsden was interested in from the farmer who grew it to the East African entrepreneur who stole it for resale."

He raised his eyebrows. "Not bad," he said. "But did you establish the Hamil connection?"

"That's the next thing," I said.

He smiled the knowing white smile. "Maybe I can help," he said. "What's the name of this entrepreneur?"

"Eugene Wollo," I said.

"Excuse me a moment." He indicated the sofa under the Rothkos. "Have a seat. If you don't like the pictures, close your eyes. I usually do."

He pulled a telephone from his pocket and wandered off across the old pine floor, a thin, elegant figure in a dark suit. I sat in the penumbra of the Rothkos. For some reason I started to think about Esias the silversmith. If you brought him to a place like this, he would think he had gone crazy. I suspected he would have liked the Rothkos, though.

Pierce came back, dropping the telephone into his coat pocket. "Man I know," he said. "Eastern African adviser to the Senate Foreign Relations Committee. We got it, I think."

"We have?" I was bewildered. I had been half drowned in corn and swamped by Rothkos. And Pierce had squared the circle with a telephone call.

"Eugene Wollo, colonel in the Sudanese police," he said. "Businessman, too. Would like government representation with the neighbors in Ethiopia. So he's making big campaign contributions to Ras Hamil's efforts." He looked down at his glass. "And I guess Rhyd Walters found out about that. And I guess a right-thinking democrat like Hamil would not have wanted his fair name smirched by the stigma of misappropriating aid. So he found a . . . solution."

So there it all was.

I smelled ashes. I felt the sun like a hot anvil on my neck, under what had once been the shade of the Alleluia Tree.

"Well," said Pierce. "I guess we should go tell the people."

26

*T*HE LECTURE GIVEN BY THE ENGLISH POET AND ORNITHOLOGIST George Devis at the house of Senator Corin Johanssen was attended by many of Lexington's most prominent citizens. That was undoubtedly the golden sentence hovering in the mind of the white-haired biro-sucker sitting on the right-hand side of the front row, just underneath the dais. Somebody had draped the lectern in a white ensign, to which I was not entitled.

There were the usual drinks before, and the usual skeletal women and their glassy-eyed checkbook caddies. Over the heads of the crowd I saw another head, thrust forward above barn-door shoulders, lit by electric blue eyes that came and went among Mongoloid creases of flesh. Poliakoff.

The crowd eddied as he forged his way toward me. His handshake was big and warm as a quilt. "My dear boy," he said in his Mitteleuropean rumble. "My dear boy."

Pierce was keeping station like a destroyer riding shotgun on an aircraft carrier. He winked. I was aware of the solidity of Poliakoff, the power radiating from him the way heat radiates from a big rock after nightfall. Prizefighters and religious maniacs would look weak and insignificant next to him.

He said, "Pierce tells me you have been having some success in pursuit of a certain person."

I said, "We're adding it up."

"But you have pieces missing?"

I shrugged. I did not know how much Pierce had told Poliakoff.

He took me by the arm and drew me close, so I was pinned away from the crowd. "I have been giving this matter some thought," he said. "As I think Pierce has told you, Mr. Hamil is a customer of one of my companies, as well as a public enemy. *Entre nous,* my analysis is that an exclusive on Mr. Hamil's arrest and indictment for first-degree murder will be as beneficial to my news interests as any deal National Dynamics may do with him." He laughed his subsonic laugh. "National Dynamics is a . . . defense industries corporation I own, which is seeking to do business with Hamil. Tough for National Dynamics stockholders, maybe. Let's hope they all have hedges in my communications corporations." He grinned, the great big rubbery grin that focused the emanation of power until it would have been no surprise if the curtains had caught fire.

He moved away. Pierce coughed, a small, self-deprecatory cough. He said, "This is the break. Talk to you afterward."

"Of course," I said.

My stomach was full of small birds, the way it always is before I have to talk in public. Mrs. Senator Corin Johanssen had fallen in alongside. She had turned upon me a couple of million candlepower of dental work. Together, we walked toward the dais.

Up I went.

They were sitting on their little gold chairs and their circular tables, the bald heads gleaming like rocks in an ice-blink of diamonds. Mrs. Senator Corin Johanssen explained that I was a very significant British person who had been sunk south of Cape Sable for the good of the Third World, the subject on which I was about to speak. She melted away to her little gold chair. I stepped up to the lectern. The lights went down. I began.

I gave them the Alleluia Tree speech, standard model.

At the end, I could see the black arms of the tree reaching into the blazing sky. And tonight there seemed to be more to say, after the place where I usually finished.

"Now, there is fire in the hills," I said. I said it quietly. The room was quiet, too. "It is the fire that came down on Rhydian Walters and my sister, his wife, and made their children orphans. But we are moving to put out that fire. We are going to bring the sword of justice on to the fire-raisers. We are going to make the hills run water, so they will never burn again. And in these newly fertile hills, we will sow—with your help —the seeds of new Alleluia Trees, so the brown lands will be green, and the people can prosper and be happy in their shade."

I stood there. The room was full of an icy silence. Bloody hell, I thought. Over the top, Devis. You've blown it.

Then the noise began.

I suppose it was only a polite clapping. But by the standards of the drawing rooms of New England, it was a volcanic eruption. I did not want to grin at them, because what I had been talking about was not a grinning matter. So I ducked my head and shoved my hands into my pockets. And suddenly the enormous head and shoulders of Serge Poliakoff were wading toward me and up on to the stage. I felt my hand yanked out of my pocket and into the air, and the big gravel voice was roaring, "Ladies and gentlemen, Mr. George Devis and PloughShare!" In a lower voice, he said, "You fixed the bastards. Grin, damn you. This is America."

I grinned. Everybody seemed to be grinning back. The jewelry was heaving like a sea swell under the sun. In the back of my mind, I heard Scotch John's voice, a sort of echo to Poliakoff's. *This is America. Assume the worst.* But I was starry-eyed with diamonds and adrenalin, and I was not listening to inner voices.

Stupid, really.

Poliakoff led me off the stage. He said, "That was fine." He sounded as if he meant it. "I want you to know that between us, you and me and my organization, we are going to nail this Hamil. Ask questions. Anything you need to know, we will find." His eyes shifted. *"Good* evening, Senator. I want to talk to you about Nicaragua." And he was gone.

Pierce looked after him and sighed. He said, "This person is a management nightmare."

I said, "He seems convinced."

Pierce smiled. He said, "We're all convinced. You've done a great job. Now you had better go pry some money out of people."

It was not until an hour and a half later that I managed to extricate myself from the throng and load myself into a taxi. I sat there and wondered how Poliakoff could help more than he had helped already. I thought: You should have gone at him with a list of questions. Make one tonight, I thought. After the boys have gone to bed. There was a wonderful homeliness about the idea. Boys safe, me belting the questions into Ricky Lee's word processor.

The taxi turned off Highway 2 and began to wind through the maples sheltering Concord, birthplace of the Revolution. The lights of houses glowed in the trees, hazed with a faint pearling of fog. "Hey," said the cabbie. "Looka dat."

Ahead was a low rise of ground covered in trees. The sky between the trunks was angry red. I knew that rise of ground. Suddenly I was not feeling smug any more. My hands were sweating, and my stomach felt as if someone had punched me in the solar plexus.

I said, "Next left." When he stopped, my fingers were shaking so badly I could not deal with the change. I spilled a handful of it through the window, tumbled out of the door and ran up the driveway, little stones crunching under the hard leather soles of my hero-lecturer shoes.

The front of the house was dark. The light was around at the back. It was a rosy flicker on the underside of the leaves. There was a little roar to it, too. I turned, looked behind me. The taxi was still there.

I shouted, "Call the fire brigade!"

There was one car in the driveway, Ricky Lee's. I ran around the house.

There was a deck, with picnic chairs and a table. Big plate-glass patio doors gave access from the house. There was no glass in the patio doors any more. Instead, there were *chevaux de frise* of orange flames. On the deck in front of the windows was a table. On the table was a checked tablecloth. The side of the tablecloth was on fire. There were three places laid. On the plates were half-eaten hamburgers and pools of ketchup. Someone had knocked over a can of Coke. There was a chair lying on its back on the boards. It looked like an interrupted barbecue, except that there was no barbecue.

My heart was hammering. The sweat was pouring off me in rivers. The house looked empty. Beside the deck, flickering in the flames, was a post with an outdoor tap and a reel of hose. I turned on the tap, pulled off a tangle of hose, and shot the jet of water on to the base of the flames. I could smell my eyebrows burning, but they might as well have been somebody else's. I was thinking: Table outside, barbecue supper, special release-day treat. Nothing short of physical violence would have induced Joe and Harry to leave a hamburger half-eaten.

Nothing short of physical violence.

The jet of water from the hose plunged into the flames with a long, steady hiss. White billows of steam rose. I could smell the chemical smoke of burning furniture, and it was taking me all the way back to Ethiopia, so I could feel the sun on my head, and see the feathery drifts of ash that coiled in the wind from the hot yellow mountains.

Inside the room, the flames abated far enough for me to see the skeletons of a sofa and two armchairs. There was something leaning on the sofa. It might have been a giant champagne glass.

It was not a giant champagne glass. It was a barbecue.

It was a barbecue that someone had picked up and heaved through the patio doors without first opening them, while Ricky Lee and Joe and Harry were having their supper.

Sirens began howling in the street. There was a lot of shouting, and the flames glowed in black helmets. The fire brigade came running into the garden.

Somehow or other, the fire went out. There was a policeman there, too. He said, "You found the fire, right?"

"Right," I said. There was a buzzing in my ears and my knees were weak. Shock, I thought. Where are the boys? Where's Ricky Lee?

"The fire chief said there was a barbecue in the Chesterfield," said the policeman. "Said the glass was on the inside of the window, like somebody threw it through. Would you know anything about that?"

"No," I said.

The policeman peered at me closely. His breath smelled of garlic. "You bin drinking?" he said.

"No," I said. "I'm English." He nodded. That would explain it. I said, "There were some people here. A woman and two children."

His radio crackled. He turned away. It was dark. The only light was the pale radiance that crawled between the trunks of the maples. Out there in the zebra-striped shade, a figure was moving. It moved hesitantly, as if walking was a new idea to it. Its knees looked double-jointed. My stomach rolled. Where the head should have been, the shoulders ran across in a straight line. I was back there on the gray sea, in the hot rain of Bill Marsden's blood, hearing the horrible plunge as his severed head hit the water.

The figure lurched. Suddenly it had a head. It had been hidden, bowed below the line of the shoulders. I walked over to it on knees that wobbled. I smelled her perfume before I recognized her. It was Ricky Lee.

She said, "Get rid of the cop." Her voice was thick and blurred.

I said, "Where are the boys?"

She leaned against me. She said, "Get rid of the goddamn cop."

The cop was leaning against the clothesline support, talking into his radio. I said, "I've found the lady whose house it is. It was an accident."

"Sure," said the policeman. The radio was spewing electric gibberish into the night. "Listen, we'll have someone come around and take a statement. Can you take care of things?"

"Sure," I said.

The firemen were bustling to and fro. One of them said, "We've damped her down. Kinda messy. Maybe you need someone to secure the place." He flipped a card out between his fingers. "My brother-in-law. Real reliable guy. D'you want me to call him from the truck?"

I said, "Thank you."

The policeman left. The firemen left. Ricky Lee was sitting on a wrought-iron seat. Her head hung forward. She said, "They took away the boys."

"Who?" I said.

"Seen him before," she said. Her voice sounded strange, as if her tongue was too big for her mouth.

I said, "Was it the deacons?"

She leaned sideways, over the arm of the seat. I heard the sound of her being sick. "Hit on head," she said when she could talk.

A truck pulled into the driveway. Someone climbed out and shone a flashlight on the side panel. The lettering said GOLDMAN GLASS AND SHUTTER. I told him to get on with it, then carted Ricky Lee into her car. "Where's the hospital?" I said.

"Not hospital," she said. Her voice was strong. "Doctor. It was the guy from Cleveland."

"Cleveland?"

"Guy with the guy hit John. He came with a process server. Two cars. Process server handed me something, left. The Cleveland guy grabbed the boys. Handed them over to someone in the car." She was crying. "I couldn't stop him. I tried. He . . . threw me at something. I can't remember any more." She was fumbling in her pocket. "Here."

She handed me a white envelope. It bore her name and my name. I ripped it open, read it by the interior light of the car. It was a court order for the return of Joseph and Henry Walters to the care and control of their guardian Sarah Ebden.

So the guys from Cleveland were minding process servers now, as well as looking for tapes and burning down houses.

I was feeling sick. I said, "Court order's one thing. Kidnapping and arson, you use the police."

She said, "He said if we called cops, boys were gone for good."

Despite the warm evening, I was icy cold.

Ricky Lee's doctor lived four houses up the road. He opened the door in his dressing gown.

"Concussed," he said. "Not badly. Rest, right?"

"Send the bill," said Ricky Lee.

"No chance, honey," said the doctor. "You the guy from the TV? She was talking about you."

I assisted Ricky Lee into the night. I drove. I did not know where I was driving. I said, "The guy from Cleveland."

"Yeah," she said.

"One of Warren Diglis's men."

"That's right."

The boys were missing, courtesy of someone who had tried to bury me alive. I wished to know where they were, and why. My stomach was tight as a walnut with nerves.

I said, "Where does Warren Diglis live?"

"Dunno," she said. "I know where he works, though."

I said, "Will your head hold out?"

She nodded. She groaned. I hated to hear her groan.

There was nothing to do but wait eight hours or so. It felt like a life sentence.

"You get some sleep," I said. "Then we'll go and find them."

27

WE CHECKED INTO A MOTEL SOMEWHERE IN THE OUTER CAM-
bridge sprawl. I called information. Then I lay on my bed and
looked at the acoustic tiles on the ceiling and tried not to think
about how the boys must be feeling. I told myself: Nobody
hurts children. But I kept thinking of Gerard and Jackson,
laughing as I fought for breath in the grain elevator. And from
there I went on to Sarah. I believed in the court order. I was not
so sure I believed in Jackson and Gerard handing the boys over
to their legal guardian.

I dozed fretfully until the light was gray outside the thin
curtains. Then I showered, in an unsuccessful attempt to get
the fog out of my head and the sand out of my eyes. I stumbled
out into a thick, drizzly morning, full of the whine and hiss of
big trucks on the road.

I extracted two cups of coffee-colored fluid from the machine
and hammered on Ricky Lee's door. She mumbled something,
unlocked the door and let me in. She was wearing a long
T-shirt. Her face was pale, the freckles gray pencil marks on
the white skin. There were dark hollows under her eyes. She

put her face into the coffee like a Bedouin putting his face into a well. I said, "How's the head?"

She smiled warily. "Good enough for rock and roll." She shook four Tylenols out of a bottle on the bedside table. "I'll be right out."

I waited in the car, watching the windscreen wipers. She came out twenty minutes later. She was walking well. When I suggested breakfast, she nodded. We ate French toast and drank a lot more coffee in a grease-fogged diner. She was all right.

There was a question on my mind. I said, "How did they know where to come looking for the boys last night?"

She shrugged. "Maybe they knew I was helping you out. Maybe they looked me up in the phone book." Her eyes shifted to the plastic-coated menu card. She did not seem interested. I put it down to her head.

I paid for breakfast. We climbed back into the car. Ricky Lee piloted me down the streaming roads toward South Boston. I stopped at a Korean store and bought her a cheap tape recorder and a notebook.

"Make a left," she said. "Down there."

I drove into a small, dirty street of pool halls and sex shops. A black man wearing ocelot-skin cowboy boots and leather peg-top trousers came out into the drizzle from under a grubby pink marquee that said PUSSYCAT CLUB. The woman on his right arm was arguing with the woman on his left arm.

"Park," said Ricky Lee.

I parked.

"Over there," she said.

There was one good window in the street. It was made of mirrored plate glass, with a black boxing-gloved fist in the middle. It was the design Jackson had worn on his T-shirt outside Sullivan's house and at J. J. Birdman's. So I would know who I was tangling with, and be fearful. The other windows in the street ran to bars and grills, protection against the brickbats of the disaffected. The silver window was unprotected. The lack of protection gave it a confident look. The neon scrawl over the top said WARREN'S. The window said that you would have to be very disaffected indeed to tangle with Warren.

My stomach felt queasy. I said, "Would you rather not do this?"

She mustered up a grin, thin-lipped but just about recognizable. "Someone torched my house," she said. Her voice was thin and nervous. "I owe it to my insurance company to visit this guy. Plus don't patronize me."

I said, "Sorry."

She said, "Do not mention it." She smiled again. This time it looked better. She leaned over in the seat, hooked my neck over in the crook of her elbow. "Good luck, podner," she said. "I like you, you know that?"

"Snap," I said.

"What does that mean?"

"Me too," I said.

"It won't last," she said. "You'll see." She was looking grim and matter-of-fact. "Let's do this."

So we climbed out of the car and walked across the road to the gym with the silver window.

I pushed the door open. Rap music rolled out like the hammer of a diesel. There was a flight of steps, done in heavy red carpet. At the top of the flight was a desk. It looked like a ladies' hairdresser's. But instead of pictures of well-prinked models, there were prizefighters, bare fists raised to guard their faces. Instead of a chic receptionist, there was a black man with a pillbox haircut, built on the general lines of a block of flats, wearing a chunky gold ID bracelet and filing the little fingernail of his left hand.

I walked up to the desk and gave him my name. I said, "I'd like to see Mr. Diglis, please."

The receptionist was not a smiler. He said, "Have a seat," and pressed an intercom switch with a salami-sized forefinger. I did not sit down. I went and looked at one of the pictures on the back wall.

It was of a white boxer after a fight. He was wearing a big silver belt. He was bleeding heavily from the brow ridges, and his nose was split. The silver plate underneath the picture said KID EPSTEIN.

I knew him better as Jackson.

When I turned around, Ricky Lee was looking at the picture too. She was even paler than earlier.

A girl came into the reception area. She had flawless skin the color of Swiss chocolate, the bone structure of Queen Nefertiti and fire-engine-red lipstick. She said, "Mr. Diglis will see you now."

We followed her through a door into a gym. The music was louder there. Two pairs of heavily padded boxers were thumping each other. Five more men were occupied with punchballs and speedbags and pieces of machinery I could not identify. There was a smell of Brut and sneakers.

The girl opened a door. There were more stairs behind the door, polished wood. At the top of the stairs was another door. The smell of sneakers was replaced by an expensive hint of Havana cigar. We walked into a small office with a blond oak desk. Certificates of some kind hung on three of the walls. In the center of the certificates was a signed photograph of Haile Selassie, late Emperor of Ethiopia. The fourth wall was made of plate glass, like the window of a recording studio. Below the window, the fighters were soundlessly laying into the machinery and each other.

Warren Diglis was behind the desk. He was reading what looked like a boxing magazine. His iron-gray hair lapped over the collar of his cream silk shirt. A Romeo y Julieta fumed in the corner of his mouth.

I said, "Mr. Diglis."

He looked up. His narrow eyes were entirely without expression. He looked like one of his fighters coming out of a corner, sizing up the opposition. He said, "Yeah."

I said, "George Devis. We've already met. And this is Ms. Klaasen."

Diglis said, "Maybe I could have some idea of what this visit is all about?"

I said, "Two men. One of them's a fighter of yours, name of Kid Epstein. The other is called Gerard."

Diglis said, "What about them?"

"Burglary. Attempted murder. Now kidnapping."

Diglis reached for his telephone, dialed a number without taking his eyes off me. He said. "Is Mr. Green there? Well, you tell him get around here soon as he comes in." He put the telephone down, pressed the record button of a tape recorder on the desk. "Mr. Green is my lawyer," he said. "You won't mind me recording this?"

Ricky Lee said, "We're all making recordings."

"So go ahead," said Diglis.

I said, "In Quogue, Maine, Mr. Epstein stole a funeral urn."

"Funeral urn," said Warren Diglis. He took his cigar out of his mouth and examined it carefully.

"In Cambridge, Massachusetts, he assaulted me."

"He did."

"In Cleveland, Ohio, he knocked me into a grain elevator. In Concord, Massachusetts, he kidnapped my nephews and set fire to the house of Ms. Klaasen."

"Fascinating," said Warren Diglis. "And why has he done these things?"

I said, "You are on record as wishing me silent."

Warren said in a low, dangerous voice, "I wish you silent, I don't come at you, what, three times. I kill you *daid.*" I believed him. "Listen here, Davis," he said.

"Devis," I said.

"Whatever," he said. "I get the feeling that you are *persecuting* me. I got the feeling first time I heard about you that maybe you do not like black people. I get the feeling that you are a *racist,* Mr. Davis Devis or whatever the hell you call yourself. I get the feeling when I have seen you on TV that you are asking a lot of people who think *Gone with the Wind* is their granddaddy's home movie to accept the idea that the British Empire is still hanging in there."

"Rubbish," I said.

"Rubbish," said Warren in what he seemed to think was an English accent. "Let me tell you something. You think you can get up there on TV with all them rich folks and tell the nation what heroes your sister and this cracker Rhyd Walters were. But I got friends, too." He waved a pug-knuckled hand at the Haile Selassie portrait. "I been looking after the interests of Ras Hamil, because I have a big and long admiration for the history of the Ethiopian people. Ras Hamil a brother."

I said, "So you steal back the evidence that Ras Hamil has committed murder."

He looked straight at me with his flat, blank face. He said, "I don't know what you're talking about."

I said, "Your man Epstein came to my boat and stole evidence."

He made a cutting gesture with his big, flat hand. He said, "You giving me and my people problems, I am going to give you and your people problems. So you can feel what it like. And so you know I know where I can put my hand on those kids, just in case you give me any more problems, and I need to persuade you 'bout something. You understand me?"

His eyes were cold as brown ice. I found I was holding my breath.

"So," he said. "I call Miz Sarah Ebden. Offer her my cooperation and assistance. I suggest that given your unruly nature she may need my assistance in enforcing the judgment of the court." His face wore an expression of quiet satisfaction, like the face of a crocodile in a mortuary.

I said, "How did you know where they were?"

Diglis said, "I read the papers."

"The papers?"

He spun a newspaper across the green leather top of his desk. It was a copy of yesterday's Boston *Echo*, folded back on itself at page five. "SEA HERO SPRINGS BOYS," roared the headline on the bottom right-hand corner. It was a detailed account of our hijacking of Joe and Harry from Greenbank, and our hauling of them down to Concord, Massachusetts. There was plenty of family background. There were quotes from me.

The byline was Ricky Lee Klaasen.

I could hear the blood roaring in my ears. Ricky Lee's face was the color of speckled paper. Her eyes were agonized. She said, "I didn't think it would matter. I thought the publicity would *help*."

Diglis had opened a file and was reading it. He made a note in the margin. His hand moved to a button on his desk, pressed it. "Well," he said. "Nice as this has been, we all have our work to do."

Feet sounded on the stairs, big and soft as a leopard's. The door opened. The block of flats from the reception desk padded into the room. I said, "Listen. You've got this wrong. This Hamil's a thief. He's been stealing from his people. He's a murderer."

Diglis said, "You get this between your ears. There have been bad days in Ethiopia. Those days are gone." He gestured at the signed photograph of Haile Selassie on the wall. "I have been a personal friend of Ras Tafari, Emperor of that country. I have to do what I can for that country now it is out from under the Stalinist jackboot. Take him out of here, Ishmael."

Something as big and hard as a crane bucket clamped on my shoulder. I twisted away. I was looking straight into the receptionist's eyes. His hand came out again. I batted it off. Something thudded into the side of my face. The world turned red and my knees buckled. I heard a high noise. It was Ricky Lee. She was going for the receptionist's throat, fingers clawed. Brave, I thought, though I knew there was something wrong with the thought. Then we were close together, being clattered downstairs into music and the smell of sneakers, and down the red-carpeted steps, and on to the sidewalk.

The sidewalk was wet and gritty on my face. There was some kind of dirt in my ear, and my head was ringing. My nose was hurting, a dull, hard throb. Someone was pulling me up. Ricky Lee.

"You're bleeding," she said.

I remembered why I did not like her. "So call your paper," I said. "Tell 'em. Sea hero thrown out of Diglis office."

"Don't," she said.

"Why not?" Blood was streaming from my nose, curling into the puddles in the gutter. "It's not a great story. But then nor was turning in Joe and Harry."

She said, "It's my job."

I said, "Then stay away from me."

"Please," she said.

"Get into the car."

I staunched the blood with Kleenex. I drove around until I saw a Hertz office. I climbed out. She said, "Where are you going?"

"Somewhere you don't get written about in newspapers."

She turned crimson behind the freckles. "I didn't *know*," she said. "I thought you were a hero. You wanted publicity. I thought you'd be *pleased*."

I said, through the window, "You're the hero."

She drove away, back to her career. The crowd on the pavement flowed around me in the gray morning.

I stood with my hands in my pockets and watched her car hiss away down the wet road.

Go to hell, Ricky Lee, I thought. You have used me as a springboard for your career. You have calculated it every step of the way. You told Diglis I had the urn. You told him I was going to visit Sullivan. You told him I was likely to be in Cleveland. And you told him where the boys were, so he could use them as a lever. Ricky Lee, I thought, you have worked me over good and proper, to hang on to your job on the Boston *Echo*.

And I miss you already.

In the Hertz office they looked hard at my wet and dirty clothes, but rented me an Escort. I clambered in and began to grope my way out of the wet gray antheap of Boston.

I stopped at a pay phone off 94 and called George Caziris.

"Yeah," he said.

I said, "They took the boys back. They got a court order."

"Yeah," he said. "Ricky Lee just called. She seemed real upset. Interesting."

"How?"

"They haven't taken them back to Greenbank. I checked. It's reasonable. They were kind of out on a limb with that anyways. They'll be under the direct care and control of Sarah Walters Ebden, I guess."

"Can I see them?"

"Not unless she wants you to. Do you want me to go to work on this?"

"Yes. Thank you."

"It's what I do," said Caziris.

28

*I*T WOULD BE NO USE DRIVING UP TO BETHEL BAY AND HAMMERING on the front door. At best, Sarah could tell me that she was within her rights as a guardian to deny me access. At worst, Chuck would blow a hole in me. Even if Chuck did not start shooting, one telephone call from Sarah to the police would give me a lot of explaining to do.

But I wanted to see the boys.

That fitted in with another idea. I turned north on 95 and headed for Quogue.

The rain stopped. The sky cleared to a crisp, bright blue. *Halcyon* was sitting out there on her mooring, good as gold, next to the lobster boats in the harbor. Peace hung over the wooden houses like a glass dome over a wedge of cheese. The gulls sitting on the posts looked at me, yawned lackadaisically, and flapped into the sky.

I looked quickly up and down the quay. Nothing moved except the gulls settling back on to new pilings. I walked between the puddles to Rooney's, leaned up against the windows and peered through the crack between the gingham curtain and the window frame. Danny was standing in the bar, the SCHLITZ sign making red reflections in his hair. There was nothing else in the bar except the furniture.

I went in.

"Hey," said Danny. "Howya doin'?"

I told him I was fine and that I had come to collect the mail.

"Sure," he said. He shoved a small pile of envelopes across the bar. "Popular guy. Lady phoned earlier. Miss Klaasen. She wanted to talk with you?"

I said, "I'll call her sometime."

Danny chuckled, a sound like glue flowing into a drain. "Sure," he said, his tallow-colored face wreathed in a big, jolly grin. "Not right now, huh? She wasn't the only one."

"She wasn't?"

"Trooper Florence wants you too. He's bin lookin' since yesterday."

"John told me."

"'S okay," said Danny. "He's gone home to his dinner about now."

"What's the forecast?"

"Fair," said Danny. "Winds light westerly, some fog, no precipitation. Why?"

"I'm going sailing."

"That's what I'd do, if I wuz you," said Danny. "Where you goin'?"

"Bahamas," I said. "Maybe Norway." I picked up the letters and left, accompanied by his wheezing laughter.

Halcyon's dory was bobbing patiently at the end of its painter. I ran down the steps, cast off, and pulled out to the boat. The engine started first twist of the key with a sewing-machine whirr and the merest wisp of black smoke. Over on the corrugated-iron superstructure of John's tug, a head appeared. I waved. The head waved back. I cast off the mooring pennant, walked aft and pushed the engine lever to ahead. *Halcyon*'s nose swung toward the tug. I went alongside. John cakewalked along the narrow side deck.

"Where you been?" he said.

I said, "Can you come sailing?"

"Now?" he said.

"Right now."

He gazed at infinity across the ramparts of his beard. He nodded, and ran into what might once have been the front door of someone's holiday cottage. I could hear the bump and clank of the Grateful Dead from within. The music stopped. He came lumbering back carrying a ragged set of oilskins in one hand and a bag in the other, and stepped over the lifelines. I put the nose for the harbor entrance and shoved the throttle forward. He said, "Where we headed?"

I said, "Up the coast a little."

I got the sails up: main, foresails and mizzen. She leaned over to starboard and began to pull a long, low snarl from the gray water. The air found its way to the bottom of my lungs, and my semicircular canals took comfort from the fact that there was something underfoot that was not concrete. Mary Morpurgo, I thought. Ricky Lee Klaasen. Nothing lasts.

We slid up under Quogue Island. I made up the sheets as John took us around the buoy and started the second part of the dogleg toward the open sea. The quay and clustered houses of Quogue drifted behind the headland. The world emptied out. Now there were only rocks and trees to port and starboard, with a hazy blue slot of horizon ahead.

"We'll anchor up for the night," I said. "Where?"

"Duck Harbor," said John.

Isle au Haut glided past against the darkening sky. We turned to port in the face of a breaking ledge. The bowsprit slid into the trees. John shuffled forward. The anchor went down with a roar. *Halcyon* dug in, and settled back into the center of the little slot in the rocks. It was suddenly quiet, except for the roar of the ledge and the wind in the trees.

I went below, put the kettle on the stove, and sat on the berth. The kettle hissed, began to whistle. John came below. I made tea. It was all quiet and normal, the way things are on a boat when people are not decapitating your crew with machine guns and ramming you. I sat down there and tried to stop thinking. It worked, the way it always does. After a while, the shaking stopped, and the hum and gibber of the mind quieted. I heard the scream of a gull outside. Bonaparte's gull, I thought. I was human again.

Until I started on the mail.

I started with the biggest envelope. It contained a folder with a gold-blocked Planet Earth surmounted by the intertwined initials PKC. Poliakoff Communications. I opened it. I started to read.

There was a note from Pierce Rapaport. It said, *Serge asked us to send you this.* The note was pinned to a sheaf of typewritten sheets and photocopies of reports. Some of the reports bore numbered superscriptions, as if they might have been government documents.

Essentially, it was hard confirmation of the story John had told me in the car on the way back from Cleveland. The isotope marking had been dreamed up by the Emergency Resources Bureau in cooperation with the CIA. A document with SECRET stamped across the top discussed wheat growers likely to be sympathetic to such a move.

There was a file on Bruno Wanamaker. Gunboat navigator, Goldwater Republican, easy mark for anything that was likely to turn patriotism into money. He had links with the CIA already. It had been easy to irradiate the wheat, pass it into the system. Other reports claimed that the object of the irradiation had been straightforward: to nail Ras Hamil (on whom there was also a dossier) in possession of filched aid corn passed on by Wollo. When the facts became public, went the argument, Hamil's name would be associated not with democratic campaigning, judged by whatever the standards of an evolving Ethiopia might be, but with theft and corruption. International agencies would find this hard to take, and Ethiopia was likely to have a lot to do with international agencies for the foreseeable future. And an Ethiopian electorate, should such a body ever come into being, would not take kindly to such a jeopardizing of the aid safety net.

There was some background. Ras Hamil commanded a small but effective guerrilla army, the ETLF. The ETLF's allegiance seemed to have changed on numerous occasions. There were, however, fixed points. After each battle and confrontation, the ETLF had emerged stronger and better armed. Every time the ETLF became stronger and better armed, Ras Hamil gained in personal power. He was now, the PKC report concluded, at the point where he was being taken seriously as a force in a new democratic Ethiopia, if such an entity should ever come into being. Failing this, he was reckoned to be tough enough to shoot his way to the top and rule by force of arms.

He was, the report concluded, a thoroughly unscrupulous slab of damnation. In the *realpolitik* of East Africa, he was a personality to be taken into account—particularly because he had falsely projected himself as populist and anti-authoritarian. The marked grain had shown that his associates were embezzling emergency aid for his benefit. But he had reached a level of authority where such trivial matters could no longer be held against him. He was too powerful to touch; regrettably, even PKC was being forced to deal with him.

Until someone stood up and showed the world what he was all about. As Rhyd had been poised to do, having as I had demonstrated got hold of a sample of irradiated corn from a Hamil handout and passed it on to Bill Marsden. But Rhyd was silenced. And so was Bill.

So far, said the final memo in the folder, I had done a great job, and presented a fair and even view of Mr. Hamil. Mr. Hamil, I probably knew already, was on a visit to the United States. He had been on the West Coast, but was due East in a couple of days. Mr. Poliakoff, in deference to the expectations of the shareholders of National Dynamics, would have to present an appearance of cooperation with Mr. Hamil. He was relying on me to balance the situation by attacking hard and continuously in my public appearances. I was referred to a list of dates and events in the file, detailing atrocities committed by Ras Hamil. PKC was committed to assist me in any revelations I felt impelled to make. It was a matter for regret that the facts in the above documents did not yet constitute adequate grounds for indictment of Hamil under U.S. law, but he was convinced that I would find a way of filling in the gaps. The memo was signed Pierce Rapaport, pp Serge Polia-koff.

Filling in the gaps.

The tape filled in a little gap. So did the flour: parts one and two. But the Ethiopian story was all assumptions and briefing document.

Except that I had an idea, involving Chuck Ebden. Call it part three.

I shoved Bill's tape into the player. There was "Birdman in the Corn," "Mr. Coffee." And the extra verse to "The Alleluia Tree."

> When the Book of Life is written
> To which this is the key,
> The Lord will post it in the library
> By the Alleluia Tree.

I tucked the papers back into the envelope, slid it behind the chart table, and pulled out the spiral-bound book of charts.

Bethel Bay was a dent at the end of a seven-mile tongue of sea that licked north between two spines of hills. Halfway down the tongue was a scatter of rocks, the biggest perhaps fifty yards across, the smallest an unjudgeable asterisk on the page. The depths around the rocks hovered between three and six feet. There were the rococo curlicues of tide rips and whirlpools. Someone, probably Rhyd, had written in pencil *bad holding*. If you got in there and got into trouble, there was no way you could drop the hook and have a think. There were no lights and no landmarks.

But there was a guide. On the chart, someone had marked a

line of bearing in faint pencil. It started by the Butcher Island light, skirted the rocks, and arrived at a little pool of two-fathom contour line. There were two transits. In daylight, with good visibility, the transits would mark changes of course. Rhyd's hand, from beyond the grave. The world seemed to be full of the works of Rhyd's hand from beyond the grave.

I climbed into the sleeping bag. John was already snoring in the forepeak. When I awoke the sun was well up, and John was cranking the anchor windlass. By the time I went on deck, *Halcyon* was creaming past the breaking reefs of the southeast corner of the Isle au Haut. I said, "Have you ever been into Bethel Bay?"

John was sitting on a cockpit locker, steering with a bare foot on a spoke of the wheel, his beard whipping in the breeze. "Sure," he said.

"Can we get in at night?"

"We can try."

I took the wheel. *Halcyon* was a live thing, the pull of her wake hard but delicate on the rudder.

John said, "Why d'you want to go by boat?"

"It's quiet."

"You shoulda cycled." He crouched in the bottom of the cockpit, out of the wind, and began to roll himself a cigarette. "At night," he said. He lit his cigarette and sighed smoke out of his black beard. "It's a bitch."

Not as much of a bitch as bicycling along a rough track with a dead-eyed moron putting Mannlicher slugs in you.

We looked at the chart and plotted a course. John banged a tape into the stereo and we cracked the sheets and broad-reached on northeast, towing a plume of white foam, "Dark Star" thundering out of the cockpit speakers. Ornithologically, it should have been interesting. There were plenty of shear-waters and petrels, and some families of sea duck engaged in low-altitude maneuvers. But there was too much else to think about. At ten-thirty in the evening, I picked up a white flash across the black heave on the port bow. An hour later, *Halcyon* was sliding past the creamy flare of waves breaking below the squat white pepperpot of the Butcher Island light. I put the nose onto Rhyd's bearing and held it there. We surged on, wake roaring, into the pit of blackness that was Bethel Bay.

29

*I*T COULD ALMOST HAVE BEEN FUN. WE HAD A BEARING, BUT A bearing is not much good if there is an unknown quantity of tide against you. The tables said the tide would be ebbing, but refused to specify how fast, except that it was between one and three knots. Since we had the tide on the port bow, that gave a possible error of two miles, which in a bay three miles wide was not very helpful. Rhyd had not believed in electronic position-finding equipment. So I steered, and John sat below, hunched over the chart and the sounder, following a line of soundings up toward the rocks. After a while, the soundings began to add up, and I became more confident.

Eventually, John clattered on deck. He said, "We better use this thing." He waved a bulky object in the blackness. Some things that might have been wires dangled from it. He fiddled in the cockpit control panel. "Searchlight," he said. The night turned brilliant white.

A white bar flicked into the haze ahead and settled on the sea. There was a long, slow heave to the black water. In the far fringes of the beam, something showed white, then faded away. And again. A rock, tearing the flank out of a swell.

"There," said John.

"Which one is it?"

"The first one," said John.

Fleetingly, I was aware of the bigness of the things riding on me. Not just the machine of wood and rope and sailcloth; but the human machine, the boys down there on the dark farm, Ricky Lee wherever she was, Rhyd and Camilla and Bill, Ras Hamil.

Unless I drove *Halcyon* into a rock.

John kept going with the light. "Pole," he said.

"What?"

"Pole." He was shining the searchlight past the white patch. Another patch swam into view, like a fried egg with a lump of gray rock instead of a yolk. On the gray rock was an upright beacon that might once have been painted white. John picked up a bearing compass. He said, "Leave that one close to starboard. Then steer 350 degrees."

My shoulders were suddenly slippery with sweat. The seas in the rocks boomed like gunfire above the rustle of the wake. We slid by.

"Whee," said John. There was an unsettling amount of relief in his voice.

"Well done," I said. There was very little relief in mine. Getting through unlit rocks at night in bad visibility and an unknown quantity of tide had been the easy part.

We anchored around the point from Bethel Bay proper and lowered the dory over the side. The tide made glucking noises under the overhangs of the hull. There were a couple of lobster boats on moorings; no yachts. I climbed down into the dory and pulled out the oars. I said to John, "Stay here."

John had lit an oil lamp in the cabin. I began to row for the shore, keeping the light astern. Five minutes later, the dory's bow hit weed.

I allowed myself one inspection with the flashlight. Then I stumbled up the rocky beach, sliding on mats of bladder wrack, towing the dory by its painter. I dragged it above the high-tide mark, turned it over and wedged it against a rock, where its bottom would look like another rock. Then I started off down the shore.

The map had shown a long, boulder-strewn beach, then a point, then the beach in Bethel Bay proper, running around to the mouth of the stream that trickled behind the farm barns. The beach was difficult in the dark. I fell once, walloped my shoulder on a rock. I pulled myself up, moved on until the spine of the headland lay across my path, deep black against the lesser black of the sky. Something above my head was trying to be a star, struggling against the roof of haze.

I went over the headland by touch, slowly, so as not to make a noise. On the far side I crawled down to the beach. Though I had never been here before, the sounds were familiar. There was the small *crunch* of wavelet on shingle; the hiss of wind in the pines. Up above, on the low cliff, would be the Tabernacle and the Walterses' burial ground. Ahead, a new star spread a glow in the fog. Except that it was not a star. It was big enough for the moon, but too yellow and too square. It was a curtained window high in the gable end of a barn. Chuck's barn.

Until that moment, I had been fully occupied with the mechanics of getting ashore and arriving at the farm. Now I was here, the night was suddenly cold, and the window was full of eyes, and I was behaving like a bloody fool, and I wanted to go back.

I sat on a boulder and stared at the window. Of course there were no eyes, and the night was no colder. What was up there was my biggest responsibility in life, orphaned, brave as lions but frightened out of their wits. It was my job to rally around them and tell them not to be frightened. There was another part, too. But that did not bear thinking about yet.

I got up and headed for the corner of the barn that did not have the lighted window. I was wearing black jeans, a dark blue sweater, and sneakers. I walked around the outside of the barn, thinking about the dog. There was no sound from the dog. Thorns snagged at me. There was the smell of wet pine needles. The back wall of the barn was a long black rampart to the left. I skirted what smelled like a muck heap. Ahead, the long, low profile of farm buildings gave way to the black silhouette of a mansard roof. The house.

I walked right, remembering the first time I had been here. The boys' rooms had been in a wing out at the back. It seemed like a hundred years ago. I stepped over the pale line of a picket fence into yielding soil. The whiff of night-scented stocks rose about me. A flowerbed. The wing with the boys' room was dead ahead, Harry's window facing me, Joe's looking the other way. Joe slept like a brick. No percentage trying to wake him. Harry it was.

The window was black and blank. There were no curtains. I thought: What if they have moved them? I pulled the flashlight from my pocket, pressed it against the glass and put my thumb on the button.

The night exploded.

I found that I was the other side of the lawn, over the picket fence and in a belt of trees. Lights were coming on all over the house. What had sounded like an explosion was a dog barking. The dog. The bloody dog.

Footsteps were thumping in hollow wooden rooms. Voices were raised. There was Sarah's, and at least one man's that I did not recognize, asking what for gosh sakes was going on. And over the whole racket soared a small one, high, clear, and familiar.

"It's perfectly all right," it said. "It's poor old Loon. He didn't like the fog, so I had him in with me. He got, er, spooked." It was the voice of trainee zoologist Harry Walters.

There was a general growling of grown-up voices. Someone took the dog into the yard. I heard whimpering, and the bang of a stable door. The dog began barking, a regular, neurotic *yowf*. The fog was wet on my face, thickening. The barking stopped. I walked quietly across the lawn and tapped on Harry's window.

Then I shone the torch on my own face, quickly. The window opened. A voice said, "Gor."

I said, "Can you talk?"

"Quiet," he said. *"Brilliant* you came. Are we off?"

"Not yet," I said.

"Oh."

"Soon."

"Yes." There was a big weight of disappointment in his voice. I said, "Can we talk in the morning?"

"Secretly?"

"Secretly."

"Behind the muck heap. Ten o'clock. Go up in the bushes and we'll be there. How did you come?"

"Swam."

"Really?" For a moment his voice was on fire with the imagining of it. Then he said, *"Brilliant.* Hop off or they'll rumble us. Up into the trees by the chapel. Nobody goes there."

He caught my hand, squeezed it. His was clammy and cold. He was keeping up appearances. Poor old Harry.

I said, "Who's here?"

"Aunt Sarah, Chuck the village idiot, two deacons and Loon. Poor dog."

I said, "Sleep tight." I stumbled away into the fog.

I found a place to hide behind the Tabernacle, a little shed in a tangle of briers that must once have been a privy, and huddled down in there. Outside, whippoorwills yelled. I may have slept. Eventually the night turned gray, then paler gray. The air smelled of wet trees. The tree trunks outside the crescent cutout of the privy door made dark verticals against a backdrop of fog.

The sun would be up soon. Cautiously, I opened the door and peered out. The trees were black and dark. I walked out, along the path, down into the yard. Early birds were singing. It was four-thirty A.M. Not even farmers got up this early.

I went down the grit path, past the end of the barn, and into the yard. The yard was dark. The big maple towered into a sky whose higher vaults were already paling with the first rays of the sun.

From the animal sheds came the sound of hooves on cobbles, the grunt of a pig. Chuck's barn was silent, and so was the cart shed and the house. A little breeze stirred the topmost twigs of the big maple tree in the yard. In the woods and on the foreshore, more birds were yelling good mornings. I walked under the branches of the great tree. Inch by inch I began to examine the trunk.

In the gap between the gable of Chuck's barn and the implement shed, a block of fog turned golden orange. For a moment I could see through the branches to the bay, where a huge molten disk was floating out of the metal water. The first rays of the sun poured through the gap.

For a moment, the ground under the tree's branches was flooded with a golden light that picked out in sharp relief the roots grappling the earth like veins on the back of a hand, and limned every crevice and pimple of the tree's bark with an unearthly glow.

I stood transfixed in the crash of birdsong and the heavenly light. I was looking at the tree trunk.

The sun-limned blemishes were not all the product of old age. Some of them were too regular: as if someone a long time ago had carved something into the bark, and it had grown back, and only with the low light of the sun across it did it become visible.

It was there in an ancient script, with serifs, the wavering ghosts of letters six inches high.

ALLELUIA

The fog rolled back. The sun went out. The light became dull and gray. Every hair on my body was prickling, as if with electricity.

CLAWHAMMER

I walked back to the privy. In my head, a verse was playing.

> The Lord will post it in the library
> By the Alleluia Tree.

I sat down. I ate half a bar of chocolate.
I waited.

30

*O*UTSIDE, A WOODPECKER CLAMBERED ON A MAPLE TRUNK. I watched it feed. The privy was no worse than a lot of bird hides I had sat in. At seven-thirty, feet slapped gently on the path. I held my breath. Sarah Walters Ebden walked past. Her head was bowed, her eyes startled-looking, open the usual fraction of an inch too wide. Her hands were clasped in front of her, carrying a thick book. She looked like a woman on her way to pray for Guidance. She went into the Tabernacle. Half an hour later she came out and went back down the path.

From the yard there came the clank of buckets, a good-morning *yowf* from the dog, and Chuck's open-mouthed humming. Animal feeding noises. I stepped cautiously out of the privy and pulled the briers back over the door. The fog lay heavy over the green hummocks of the Brethren's graves, beading the lawn with moisture. Sarah Ebden's tracks were still there.

I kept to the path. *Only the Brethren may penetrate the Tabernacle.* There was a white wooden porch over an arch-topped door.

The door had a big iron latch. Slowly, I raised the latch and went in.

My mouth was dry, my palms wet. I do not know what I had been expecting. My mind was an untidy attic of bones, cabalistic symbols, visions of Judgment.

There was none of that.

There was a room of white-painted planks, with concentric rectangles of benches. The benches were of oak, with a high black polish of use and age. On one of the walls was a white board bearing the inscription WITH THEE WILL I ESTABLISH MY COVENANT. God's words to Noah, before he washed the world clean with the Flood.

Facing the inscription on either side of the door were wooden panels, floor to ceiling. At the top were ten names, each suffixed by the name *Ark* and the date 1691. One of the names was J. Walters. From the original ten names descended lines, in the manner of a family tree. The lines crossed and recrossed, marriages and intermarriages. There were a lot of dead ends. Very few new names were admitted.

I looked at the bottom of the Walters line. John Walters and his wife Rachel were shown as having one daughter, Sarah, who had married Joseph Ebden, deceased, and had offspring Charles Ebden. There was no mention of Rhydian Walters or Maria Walters. But when I looked closely, there were two pale spaces in the fudge-colored wood, as if something written there had been removed. Below the name of Sarah Walters Ebden, there was blank space waiting. Ready for Joe and Harry when they graduated from the family Bible.

I began to shiver. Not more than 120 names descended from the original ten. I wondered how many lives the Brethren had wrecked in the name of salvation.

I walked out onto the porch, closed the door softly behind me, and moved along the path and into the trees. At ten o'clock, I was waiting in a rhododendron bush by the muck heap. Feet approached, running. A voice said, "Are you in there?" Joe's voice.

"Yep."

"Great."

"Anyone watching?"

"No. We've got ten minutes. Then we're back to brainwashing."

I scrambled forward in the bush. They were wearing T-shirts and jeans. Both of them looked white, with black circles under their eyes, as if they were not getting enough sleep. I hugged them both. Joe said, "It's great to see you."

Harry said, "I already told him that."

"So," said Joe. "Can we get out of here?"

"Not as easy as that," I said. "There's a court order. They'll put me in jail if I take you away."

"Oh," said Joe.

"But in a few months, it's your turn with me."

"A few *months,*" said Joe.

"I don't know if we can hold out that long," said Harry. He looked pale and grim, most un-Harryish.

"What do you mean, hold out?" I said.

Harry said, "They keep on at you. Eight in the morning till ten at night. Grind, grind, grind."

"They're trying to make us say we don't want to go back to England," said Joe. "And they're grown-up, and we're not, so I should think we'll probably give in." He was chillingly matter-of-fact.

Harry said, "But I do want to go back." He was not matter-of-fact. He was trying desperately not to show it, but he was crying. "It doesn't matter what they make me say."

I thought about Rhyd's bloody stupid will. Work with him on music, or the village project, or the PloughShare workshop, and he would give until he turned himself inside out. Ask him about the Brethren, and he would shut up tight as a bank vault. It was beginning to look as if he had never admitted anything, even to himself. When he had made the will, he must have made it by dirty old conditioned reflex, and blagged it past Camilla. I felt a twinge of the sadness I had felt when he and she had gone away from Devon to Africa.

Jealousy.

Still, there it was in black and white, and there was no Rhyd around to argue with. All the Brethren needed was a declaration by the boys in front of a lawyer. If they got that, the boys would be stuck.

I said, "What happens here in the daytime?"

"They do farming," said Joe. "We read books and get lectured."

I said, "Does Sarah ever go out?"

Joe said, "She comes with us and those bloody deacons every afternoon for a ghastly nature ramble. Listen, we'll have to go back."

I said, "Won't be long now."

Harry nodded, not trusting himself to speak. Joe grinned at me, his artificial grin, to put me at my ease. Tears of impotent rage heated my eyes. I kissed them both.

They walked away. As they rounded the barn, Joe raised his hand in a small, cocky gesture of farewell.

I slid back into the bushes. The morning wore on.

At twelve-fifteen, Chuck came out and loaded a couple of bales of straw on to a box on the back of a tractor. When he had finished he went into the house, reemerged with a tray and took it to his barn. Lunchtime. After lunch, the boys came out onto the porch. On either side of them was a deacon, wearing the uniform of short haircut, tieless white nylon shirt buttoned at the neck, and charcoal-gray trousers. Bringing up the rear was Sarah.

I saw a brief, pale flash of Harry's face as he turned his head, unable to stop himself glancing at the bushes where I had been hiding. Then they were off, walking up the track toward the road.

I looked down through the fog at Chuck's barn. There was no movement. Carefully, I walked through the trees toward the house.

When I came to the edge of the clearing I paused and took a deep breath. I heard the tuneless humming. I stood still among the trees. Chuck stumped across the far side of the yard to the tractor. The diesel started. Gears clashed and a transmission churned. He pulled the wheel over, jounced out of the gate and around the corner in the track, the black-and-white dog lolloping after the back right-hand wheel, tongue out, tail high.

Leaving me in sole possession.

I got up. I dusted myself down. I walked over to the house, up the steps, and in at the door.

The Lord will post it in the library
By the Alleluia Tree.

I went through the house.

The only writing downstairs seemed to be in the embroidered texts on the walls. I looked in all the drawers. Apparently Sarah did not read. In a small back room there was a desk. The desk drawer held five files of papers. There were bank statements, details of farm accounts, automobile expenses and household expenses. There was also a file without a label, which held documents that dealt with financial transactions with the Brethren. They seemed to be the accounts of a low-input farm run frugally by someone not given to speculative investment. Presumably there were big capital funds in the background, because the Brethren file contained details of five-figure payments made by the Walters Trust quarterly to a numbered account in Bangor, Maine. I guessed that the Bangor account might have a lot to do with Greenbank. That would be one of the reasons why so much effort was going into the conversion of Joe and Harry. Rhyd had left a lot of money. I suspected Elder Hornbeck was at least as keen on the boys' inheritance as on their souls.

I went on through the drawers. Sewing materials; photographs; scraps of cloth. The important odds and ends of a frugal life. Nothing.

I moved on. The boys' rooms were boys' rooms, cluttered

with clothes, smelling of old socks. There was a room at the end of the corridor with a Ping-Pong table. Upstairs, the deacons had a room each. One of them had left a body-building magazine under his pillow. Sarah's room had a single bed, a threadbare carpet, bare walls. On her bedside table was the suitcase-sized Bible. Someone had once told me that Bibles were favorite places for hiding things. The Bible had a lock. The hasp was engaged, but when I pulled it with a finger it came open. There was the family tree. There were the pages, the type, the smell of damp. Nothing else. I went downstairs.

A robin was looking for grubs under the Alleluia Tree. Otherwise, nothing moved. I let myself out of the front door, and listened.

There was the sigh of a tiny breeze in the branches, the cooing of a dove. There was the crunch of waves on the beach, the grunt of a pig in the shed opposite. There was no sound of voices or tractors.

I walked under the tree to Chuck's barn.

There was a door in the end of the barn that faced away. Someone had painted it yellow and red and blue, exciting ten-year-old's colors. It was not locked.

The door led straight into a living room. It was a child's room, but wrong. There was a smell of sweat instead of socks, a set of barbells on a stand, and a pile of clothes in the middle of the floor. Against the far wall was a green enamel gun cabinet with a DANGER sticker on the door. To the right was a big stereo and a rack of cassette tapes. In the corner, next to a stuffed moose's head, was a spiral staircase. Between the uprights supporting the handrail sat a dozen or so teddy bears. There were no magazines, books or newspapers.

There was a Dexion shelving system with a TV, a line of chrome-plastic-on-marble shooting trophies, and photographs of Chuck and Rhyd: Rhyd with guitar; Rhyd teaching Chuck to shoot, both of them grinning. I found I was almost warming to Chuck.

But I did not look at the photographs. I looked at the olive-green metal of the shelf units. On the topmost cross member, someone had a long time ago painted in blood-colored gloss the word LIBRY.

By the Alleluia Tree.

Suddenly my heart was beating like a drum.

Next to the photographs was a pile of leather-bound books, large quarto size. I pulled one down and opened it. It was a stamp album. I leafed through it. There were a lot of Ethiopian stamps with recent postmarks; some British stamps too. The book was not yet half full. I could track my visits to Ethiopia from the British stamps: once a year, around about Christmas. I had brought the jiffy bags back to London, posted them airmail to the U.S.A. I looked at the last two Christmases, leafed through to this one.

Stopped dead.

Last Christmas and the Christmas before, there was one stamp. This Christmas, there were two, twice the value of the previous years. Postal charges had gone up. But the cost of airmailing a cassette to America had not doubled.

I remembered going to the post office to post them the day I had arrived back from Africa. My mind had been filled with horror and shame. I had been running on autopilot. I had handed over the bag. I had hardly known where I was. The woman behind the counter had done the stamps.

It was not postal charges that had doubled. It was the number of cassettes in the envelope. But what would have been the point of sending Chuck two identical copies of the cassette? One would be enough for his collection, and Sarah's taste in music, if any, would presumably tend to the sacred.

The Lord will post it in the library by the Alleluia Tree.

I went to the cassette rack.

There must have been three hundred of them there, each neatly in its box. It was mostly old country, Waylon Jennings and Johnny Cash and Willie Nelson. On the right-hand end was a separate rack. There, the cassettes were home-recorded. I knew what they were before I pulled out the first one: Rhyd's specials from Africa. There were twenty-eight of them, numbered, each in its case. After twenty-eight, there were five spare slots in the rack.

I flicked open the player, slotted in the number twenty-eight tape.

Die with Mr. Coffee in the sand.

It was the one I had posted from England. One of the two I had posted.

I listened to the song, flicked it forward. There was "Birdman in the Corn," "The Alleluia Tree." I stood gazing at the cassette case as if it would tell me things. Of course, it told me nothing. I was sweating now. The new verse to "The Alleluia Tree" was running in my mind. I matched the cassettes to the stamps. They were a perfect fit. Except for the second cassette from the last parcel, which was not there. Which should be there, because the other cassette, number twenty-eight, that Bill had called part two and mailed to himself at Sullivan's address, was the pointer.

The flour, part one. The Alleluia Tree cassette, part two. And part three, missing.

Drawn a blank.

I walked quietly up the spiral staircase.

The bedroom was the same size as the living room. There was a single bed and a huge wardrobe built of dark wood. Above the bed was a big poster of Rhyd wearing an Ace Logging baseball cap, hitting a chord on his Martin D45. It was a good photograph. The eyes were direct and powerful and they followed you around the room. Good afternoon, Rhyd, I thought. Nasty place you have landed up in.

The wardrobe contained a suit, a baseball jacket, some fishing rods, and a baseball bat. It smelled even worse than the downstairs room and there was nothing interesting in it. I shut it fast, explored the rest of the room. It was tidy. If there had been another cassette, I would have found it. There was nothing. I went downstairs again.

Chuck had been gone forty minutes. I was beginning to feel rushed and worried. A fly was buzzing. The sound turned into something else. A tractor, jouncing around the corner and in at the gate of the yard. The engine stopped.

There was a sash window over the stereo, looking out through the trees to the bay. I pulled it open, shoved my legs out and slid over. Perched on the windowsill, I pulled down the sash as far as I could. Then I dropped the eight feet to the ground.

The door opened and closed. The window stayed shut. I crept away, my shoulder brushing the shingles of the barn's side. At the end, I followed the stream down to the beach. The fog closed behind me like a door, shutting out the buildings. I slipped on the boulders and broke a fingernail climbing across the spine of the headland. I was hungry and tired. The boys knew I was trying to help them. I had found another Alleluia Tree, and proved to my own satisfaction the existence of another tape, which was not there. But in the end, I had achieved nothing.

The dory was where I had left it. I pulled it down the beach, rowed out into the gray pea soup. *Halcyon's* masts solidified ahead. John stuck his head out of the hatch when I hailed. I climbed aboard, dragged the dory on deck.

John said, "How'd it go?"

"Fine," I said.

"Nobody see you?"

"Nope."

"Kids there?"

"Yep."

"Shoulda brung 'em."

The same thought had been passing through my mind. But in the face of a court order, I had to do it right, or not do it at all.

"There goes the music," said John.

Fog is peculiar stuff. In fog, the sound of a horn or the bell on a buoy can seem to be coming from quite the wrong direction.

Sometimes it blots out noise as efficiently as a pair of ear protectors. Sometimes it does exactly the reverse.

Today was one of those days. We were more than half a mile away from the barn in a straight line. The music came over the gray water small but clear. It was Rhyd, as usual; Rhyd in Ethiopian mode, flatpicked guitar, mandolin and synthesizer, stripped to the bone, playing "Birdman in the Corn." This version sounded as if it had a banjo part. There was no banjo part on "Birdman in the Corn."

The wind puffed the noise away. The whinny of the starter gave way to the hammer of the diesel. I went to sleep.

The fog cleared soon after dawn. In Quogue, we picked up the mooring buoy. I took John to the tug, rowed to the quay, and trudged along to Danny's.

Danny was leaning on his bar, his face cream-colored under the Ronald Reagan hair. He brought coffee. Beside the cup he tossed a couple of envelopes held together with an elastic band. There was a letter from Pierce Rapaport, asking me to call the *Duchess of Malfi* as soon as possible. And there was a note in a big, backward-sloping hand, with Ricky Lee's name on the back of the envelope.

I called Pierce and told his secretary I would be in Boston the following morning. Then I opened Ricky Lee's.

It was an apology. I should realize, she said, that she had only been doing her job. Could I call her at the office?

I thought about Ricky Lee. She had introduced me to the PKC people, without whom none of the funds would have been raised. She had followed me doggedly halfway across America. She had pointed me at Greenbank. She had looked after the boys.

And sold us down the river.

I thought particularly about the way she had sold us down the river. It certainly did not fit as an act of malice. It was not unnatural that a probationary reporter seeking a staff job should have filed a good story. And she was not to know that it could hurt anyone.

It took some understanding. But it was understandable, if you wanted to understand it.

Another thought occurred to me, as if it had been hiding under the first thought. One of the reasons I was being understanding was that I was missing her.

I got up. I went to the telephone. I dialed the number of the Boston *Echo*.

31

*T*HE VOICE ON THE FAR END PUT ME THROUGH TO THE NEWSROOM.
A woman's voice said, "Ricky Lee Klaasen? I'm sorry, Ms.
Klaasen doesn't work here."

I said, "She does."

The voice said, "She has left us."

I said, "What do you mean, left you?"

"I'm afraid I can't discuss this, sir." She sounded like a
secretary.

I said, "Are you trying to tell me she was fired?"

"I'm not trying to tell you anything. I'm afraid I can't
discuss this, sir."

I said, "Please put me on to someone who can."

I got a new voice, a man. He said, "Can I help you?"

I said, "I'm a story of Ms. Klaasen's. Do you have a
forwarding address?"

"I don't know . . ." he said.

I said, "Ms. Klaasen was a probationer. Did she get fired?"

The voice at the end said, "Who is this?"

I gave him my name.

"Mr. Devis," said the voice in a sort of surprised purr. "Just where are you?"

I said, "I want to know about Ms. Klaasen."

"We'd like to talk to you."

I said, "So tell me where Ms. Klaasen is."

He said, "You are correct. She was fired."

"Why?"

"She refused to work on a story."

"What story?"

"A story about you. I'd like—"

"Did she leave a number?"

"I guess so."

"Would you please give it to me."

"Well . . ."

"If you want to talk to me, give me her number."

He sighed. "Tough guy."

"That's right."

There was a pause. He gave me the number. "Now," he said. "About—"

I hung up on him. Then I dialed the number he had given me.

"Hello?" said a dull voice.

"Ricky Lee?"

The voice brightened. *"George,"* she said.

I said, "You got fired."

"Oh sure," she said. "But . . ."

"Why?"

"They wanted stories I wasn't ready to write," she said.

"What stories?"

She said, "The editor's trying to turn you into a wild man. Like, the Noble Savage? Outside the law, kidnapper, all that. I wouldn't do it."

"Why not?"

"Because I know it's not true." She was silent for a long time. She said, "There is a problem, being a reporter. The only good stories are too important to write about the way you have to write about them to sell papers." She hesitated. "And there are some things that make work seem . . . not all that important. I'd like to talk to you. Not as a reporter."

"As a what?"

"Folksinger? Human being?"

I said, "I'm on my way to Boston. Lecture tomorrow."

She said, "You can pick me up from work tonight."

"Where are you?"

"Shady Grove." She gave me an address in Cambridge. "Singing till eleven."

I said, "I'll be there."

I cleaned up *Halcyon*. Over on the tug, John was watering his plants. I said, "I'm off."

He said, "I'm coming."

I said, "Sure." It was a relief. There would be reporters. And Warren Diglis's staff.

I threw my suit into a bag. John arranged for a friend of his to take us to Bangor in his pickup truck. In Bangor we collected the Mustang and headed for Greater Boston.

It was ten o'clock by the time we got in. The Shady Grove was a sort of roadhouse in a quiet inner-suburban street in Cambridge. The place was drowsy with the sound of late lawnmowers as we pulled up in the car park. John was wearing a fringed suede jacket and Kodiak boots. The bespectacled man on the door gave him a nervous look as we went in, but seemed reassured by the skull-and-roses T-shirt. Deadheads don't bite.

There was a big room with a wooden floor and tables about half full of people wearing checked shirts and drinking beer. Ricky Lee was on the stage in the lights, with a made-in-Korea Martin copy around her neck. She was wearing a black silk shirt, a sequinned waistcoat, jeans with a big studded belt, and cowboy boots. Her face stood out startlingly against the somber collar of the shirt. The eyes came across the fold-back speakers and grabbed you. If she had been the junior partner in her duo with Maria Walters, they must have been a very hot duo. The songs were wry and funny, and her voice was fine: innocent but tough, like a McGarrigle. She could play guitar, too, modified flatpicking with jazzy swing chords.

I called the *Duchess of Malfi,* left a message for Pierce. We sat down at a table near the back and ordered beers.

Pierce arrived after half a dozen songs. He sat down and ordered a Bell's, no ice. We listened to the rest of the set. When she had finished, we clapped like hell.

"Hard way to make a living," said Pierce. "She's good, though. So how's it going?"

I said, "Not bad." I did not want to admit that I was up against a missing tape and a dead end.

"Did you manage to use that material we sent?"

I said, "It was useful background. Not there yet."

He grunted. He said, "Serge wants to give you a chance to use it."

"What do you mean?"

"I'll let him tell you. He has a plan. He brought Ras Hamil over, right?"

"Of course."

"So I think he wants you to meet the guy. You can ask Hamil the questions you have to ask. You have some questions for him, I assume?"

"Of course." There was a hollow in my stomach. I grinned what I hoped was a confident grin. My case was incomplete, and Hamil did not sound like a man given to answering questions. "It's good of him to give us this much support."

Pierce smiled wearily. "Serge only supports himself," he said. "Don't you ever kid yourself otherwise. Shall we go?"

I said, "This time of night?"

"One of his little whims," said Rapaport. "I think you'll be pleased." He grinned. "At least I hope you will. I've been urging him on. I'd fit in, if I were you." Again there was something weary about the grin. "You get used to fitting in, after a while."

There was a hand on my shoulder. I looked up and saw Ricky Lee. "That was great," I said. She looked shiny and happy and slightly larger than life, the way people look when they have just come off stage. I kissed her on the mouth. She kissed me back.

Pierce said, "Sorry to hear about your job."

She shrugged. Her hair bounced around her face. "I'm freelancing again," she said. Her hand was on my shoulder. The sequins on her waistcoat sparkled in her eyes. "I guess there's not much you can do, right?"

"It's up to the editor," said Pierce. "I'll keep my eyes open." He turned to me. "We should go see Serge now, I guess." He called a waiter and paid his bill.

Ricky Lee took my hand.

I said, "You wanted to talk."

She said, "I wanted to see you." She smiled.

I felt as happy about that as she looked.

She said, "Do you have somewhere to stay?"

I said, "No." There was a sudden thickness in my voice.

"I'm at a friend's house. Girlfriend. You're welcome there."

I thanked her.

"See you later," she said. She stood on tiptoe, kissed my cheek, and went away backstage.

I said to John, "I'll go with Pierce."

John nodded. Pierce was one of the good guys.

Pierce's car was a Jaguar XJS V12, beautifully kept. We talked about tomorrow's lecture at a Hunger Brunch in the Poliakoff Center. He drove fast, but with caution. John was following on behind. I said, "There's something else."

He raised his eyebrows.

I told him about the boys. I told him about the Brethren, the levers they were applying. I said, "Is there any chance that we could get Mr. Poliakoff interested?"

He posted the Jaguar through a letterbox-sized slot between a truck and a cab. He said, "All in good time."

"Meaning not now."

Pierce said, "Have you been reading the financial pages?"

"No."

"Serge has been borrowing a lot of money. He needs a . . . feel-good factor. You're it."

"What do you mean?"

"You and he are nailing despots hand in hand. I was telling you about the . . . difficulties of running a news organization when its interests run counter to the industrial conglomerate of which it forms a part. Well, Serge has his problems with this, too. I know that he is using your . . . mission *vis-à-vis* Ras Hamil to solve these problems. On the one hand, there's you, the good guy against this bandit Hamil. On the other, there's the business Hamil might do with Poliakoff companies if he should come to power in his country. All I can tell you at the moment is that you and he and the Communications Corporation are on the same side, and Hamil's on the other. I guess Serge has made his calculations." We were waiting at a stop light. It turned green. I saw his clean-cut face pale and ghastly in the emerald glow. "You nail this guy, we all feel good, and so does the share price. A bird in the hand, George." He shrugged. "I'm afraid your nephews don't . . . fit just now." He smiled. "But we'll think of a way," he said. "Patience. One thing at a time."

Pierce knew what he was talking about. He drove to the dock where the *Duchess of Malfi* sat reflected like Brighton Pier in the black water.

The matelot at the end of the gangway recognized me. John arrived, but stayed in the car. I passed up the gangplank and into the silk-walled cabin with the Van de Veldes. Pierce said, "Whiskey?"

I nodded. He handed me a thick tumbler like a French marmalade jar, half-full. He poured himself a big one, too. It was the second drink I had seen him have this evening. Something in his eye made me think they might not have been the only ones. "Serge's on the phone," he said. "Any minute now."

We talked for perhaps five minutes about the lecture I was giving the next day. Pierce went through. After five minutes he came back with Poliakoff. Poliakoff was still speaking into a portable phone, saying what sounded like a series of elaborate goodbyes in a language that could have been Greek. He tucked the phone into his pocket, enveloped my hand in his hot, soft grip, and poured himself a slug from the decanter. The papery bags under his eyes had deepened. "So," he said. "Pierce tells me you are having a little problem with your pursuit of Mr. Hamil."

I said, "I'm getting closer. There are gaps."

He said, "I think it's time you met the old chap."

I stared at him. "Met him?"

Poliakoff smiled a smile of vast benevolence. "You won your race," he said. "An ex-Englishman's word is his bond. Let me explain. I told you I have a company named National Dynamics. Mr. Hamil has been on the West Coast, as you know. He is to visit the National Dynamics Plant on Monday, look at a gadget we have built up there. The plant's up the coast, by Portsmouth Naval Shipyard. I want to give you the chance to ask him some direct questions."

I drained the whiskey. I said, "What exactly do you mean?"

The smile widened. He said, "I have an obligation to National Dynamics shareholders, and of course myself. Mr. Hamil is apparently very impressed with this gadget. He feels it could be of use. I am under pressure from the directors and shareholders of National Dynamics to sell it, or anyway to get some polite remarks about it from . . . distinguished possible clients in this type of market. But I have a big sympathy with the human side of this, and with what you have been working on already it will make a great story." He drank, grinning as if he had explained everything in the minutest detail. "So you go to National Dynamics. And you talk to him. He'll bring a bodyguard, but you will be with my people. See what you can get. Okay? Day after tomorrow. Monday. We'll wire you for sound. You can ask him what you want to ask him in perfect privacy and safety. Maybe you can fill in your gaps."

I stared at him: the twenty stone of him, pear-shaped, the eyes glittering like sapphires in their nets of creases. I said, "What's this gadget?"

He grinned. "Wait and see," he said. "Oh, by the way. Don't worry about Warren Diglis."

"Worry?"

He smiled. "I heard he has been giving you trouble. I have had a little word with Mr. Diglis. I own a sporting events promotion corporation. The president of this corporation knows . . . facts about some contracts. I hope he will not bother you again." He raised his hands. "So," he said. "We all need our sleep. See you tomorrow at the Center. Don't wear a tie."

Attention to detail, the secret of power. I said, "I'll be there."

I left. John was waiting at the bottom of the gangway. We drove back out to Concord.

I said, "I guess you don't have a job any more."

John said, "I'll stick around."

Since her house had burnt out, Ricky Lee was staying with a friend in a leafy road. She was picking a guitar on a sofa by the window. Her friend was a dark woman with a pale, humorous Italian face. She looked nervously at John.

Ricky Lee said, "He's a nice guy."

The friend's name was Erin. She was a dancer. She seemed slightly consoled. I was not sure how much. It had been a long couple of days. I was very tired. I hung on to Ricky Lee. Her arm went around my waist. Erin was looking half-worried, half-smug, the way women look when something is working out the way they have decided it should. John said, "I kin crash on the Chesterfield." He lay down, pulled the carpet over himself, and began immediately to snore.

"Old seaman's trick," I said. I could feel Ricky Lee's shoulders shaking as she laughed.

Then we went upstairs.

CLAWHAMMER

There was a room with a polished wooden floor, a big white bed, and decoy ducks on a dressing table.

Ricky Lee came back from the bathroom. She was wearing a white nightdress, and she was smiling. She looked beautiful. I opened my mouth to tell her so. No sound came out. My eyelids crashed down. I was asleep.

32

*W*HEN I WOKE, THERE WAS A BROAD STRIPE OF SUN PAINTED ACROSS the bed from the crack in the curtains. It took me a minute to work out where I was. It was the perfume that put me straight. I turned my head and looked across the pillows. There was a dent where Ricky Lee's head should have been, but no Ricky Lee. I swung my feet out of bed, cleaned my teeth in a bathroom full of ferns and soap in the shape of exotic fruits, and went downstairs.

Erin was in the kitchen. She grinned a faintly bawdy grin. "Ricky Lee had to go work," she said. "Said to say sorry she missed you, she had to go write about somebody's collection of decoy ducks, see you tonight. You want coffee?"

I drank coffee. John had disappeared, apparently to see friends. Erin talked cheerfully about the insecurities of the journalist's life. She said, "I'm real glad Ricky Lee found you."

I nodded. "Me, too," I said.

"She's a real nice person." Erin looked at me sideways out of her long black-fringed eyes.

I said I had guessed that. Then I went upstairs and attired

myself in the shirt and suit, no tie, preparatory to addressing the Hunger Brunch of International Assistance.

This was not a gathering of rich people, waving checkbooks. This was a gathering of the converted, charity workers and contributors and Third World supporters, held in the conference hall at the Poliakoff Center off Harvard Square. I climbed into the Mustang and set off.

I was nervous, the way I was always nervous before talking to a big crowd. The Poliakoff Center was a white concrete gasometer with some conservatories attached. A girl in a short, tight skirt met me at the door. She had a bright red mouth and long red nails. "Serge is waiting for you," she said. "I'm Marlene. I type for him."

She led me backstage. Her walk owed less to the typing pool than the catwalk. I could hear the rumble of Poliakoff's voice before we got into his room. It was mostly made of glass, with a distant view of the ziggurats of downtown Boston. He was on the telephone as usual, dressed in a seersucker jacket four feet wide. He raised a hand, finished his call, and said, "So there you are," with the smile that buried the blue-chip eyes in the wrinkles. "Good crowd out there. Five thousand."

I said, "Five thousand?"

"Magic of TV," he rumbled. "Fifty-dollar tickets. Auditorium donated free of charge, rock and roll bands playing buckshee, free publicity on my stations. I provide a little snack for all. Clear your chaps a quarter of a million dollars."

"Fine," I said, dry mouthed.

"And tomorrow, you meet the man himself." He pulled a sheet of paper from a folder, handed me a laminated card. "Here's a press pass. Lets you go where you like at National Dynamics. Do you have a broadcast-quality tape machine? No? Didn't think so. You can stay the night in my hotel in Portsmouth. We'll kit you out tomorrow." He glanced at the paper. "Well," he said. "That's about all. We're very pleased with what you've done so far. I hope that you'll think of some questions for Mr. Hamil when you get alone with him." He smiled. "I hope you don't mind heights."

"Heights?"

"Didn't they tell you?" said Poliakoff. "National Dynamics is the world's foremost manufacturer of semirigid dirigibles. We're sending you and Hamil up in an airship. Just you and him and the pilot. Nice and private."

I stared at him. I could feel cool air in my mouth. I said, "Don't be stupid."

His face stiffened for a moment. Then he laughed. He said, "Ridiculous, isn't it? Mr. Hamil wants an airship. Quaint. Barbaric." Then his smile vanished and his mouth was a lipless slot, and the eyes no longer twinkled like sapphires but had the dull, poisonous gleam of copper sulfate crystals. "To you," he said. "Not to him or me or the shareholders of National Dynamics." He laid his big, competent hands on his knees. "This is a very beautiful airship," he said. "Full of computers. Nonflammable helium gas. From this one airship you can protect a thousand miles of coast against submarines. You can prospect for minerals more efficiently than from any other type of platform. You can patrol a frontier without the necessity of returning to base. This is a very versatile aircraft, Mr. Devis, and it has cost my company National Dynamics thirty-one million, two hundred and fifty thousand dollars to develop. It is a canceled contract with the U.S. government, because there are no more submarines to guard against. I think that maybe it would be useful to Mr. Ras Hamil, but more than that, I want people to *see* this thing; this beautiful, ecologically sound, gigantic thing." His voice had become Churchillian. "And I will show it to them because you are in it, you and your enemy. And once again it will catch the people's imagination. They will love to watch this airship on their television screens and hear about the meeting that has taken place on board between our British hero and the assassin of his sister and the interpreter of country songs Rhydian Walters." He raised the hands. He banged them on his knees. "You wish to talk to Ras Hamil for your reasons. I set the venue for my reasons. I am not a charitable institution. So we each achieve our goal." There was sweat on his forehead. "So," he said. "Now we understand each other." He pulled out a cigar, licked the end with a fat, gray tongue. "Now," he said. "Get out there and pitch it to 'em hard."

I said, "Of course." My mouth tasted of ashes. Ras Hamil, fine. But airships. I was not at all sure about airships.

"Well," he said, switching on the smile again, "mustn't keep you from your public."

He sailed out of the room, prodding buttons on his telephone.

"Ten minutes, Mr. Devis?" said Marlene the catwalk typist. She handed me a typewritten sheet. "Your schedule for tomorrow." She closed the door discreetly. I gazed upon the bougainvillea scaling the wall and reasoned with myself.

Over the past two weeks, Serge Poliakoff had netted Plough-Share close to a million dollars. I stared at the chair in which he had been sitting, and told myself: What you have heard is real. Not a hallucination.

I told myself several times. It did not make it much easier to believe. But I was sitting in Poliakoff's office, with Poliakoff's crowd muttering like surf behind the wall. I had to think in Poliakoff terms, like Pierce Rapaport.

That made it easier. I arrived at a state of mind where I could accept the evidence of my ears. It was up to me to make sure he got a story involving his damned airship. What I thought of his mental balance did not enter into it.

I took a deep breath, to steady my own mind. The door opened. Marlene undulated across the marble. She said, "I guess we're ready now, Mr. Devis."

I nodded. It was a bright, summery day in the conservatory, but I had the impression the sun had gone in. Don't be ridiculous, I told myself. Airships are fine. And you are not walking away now that you are this close. You have done that once already.

Then I was out in the auditorium under the bright lights and the eyes of five thousand people eating smoked salmon and scrambled eggs at Serge Poliakoff's expense. And there were other things to think about.

I moved around, talking to people as they ate brunch. I pretended to eat some myself. Then I walked on to the stage, shuffled across to the lectern, and made the speech.

It was the usual Alleluia Tree speech, and it went down a storm. By the end of it, it was as if Rhyd and Camilla were standing alongside me on the stage, and I could feel the warm glow of their approval. But I kept going after the windup.

"Tomorrow," I said. "Tomorrow, I have to meet the architect of all this misery: Ras Hamil. This is a guy who draws his campaign funds from your tax dollar and gets rich off your charitable contributions. I am going to ask him face to face what it is like to grab it all for yourself and ignore the children who are starving in the road. I am going to ask him how he can machine-gun aid workers and expect a hearing in the U.S.A. I am going to make him answer if it kills me. I am going to stop this man. Dead."

There was a quadriphonic roar of voices: well-intentioned liberal opinion, baying for the blood of the oppressor before it got down to the rock and roll and children's events.

I walked off the stage, streaming sweat. Marlene told me that had been great. Then she said, "We had a phone call for you." She handed me a mobile.

It was Ricky Lee. "Morning, lover boy," she said. "You woke up. How's it going?"

I said, "Fine. I have a date with Hamil."

She said, "That's what I'm ringing about. I'm through with the wooden ducks. You want to see some videos?"

"Videos?"

"Tapes of TV handling of your lectures. It could save you time with Hamil tomorrow." Her voice sounded guarded. "I'm at the News Actuality studios downtown. Ask for Editing Suite B."

"Couple of hours," I said. I called Erin's answering machine, left a message for Scotch John. A bluegrass band had started playing "John the Baptist" on the stage. Marlene piloted me out into the hall and started introducing me to the Poliakoff press. I looked past the camera lenses and into the crowd. I wondered if Serge Poliakoff was truly powerful enough to keep Warren Diglis away from me. I could see no boxers out there. All I could see were the faces of a lot of well-intentioned Americans on a day out with their families.

I grinned and shook hands and answered questions. At six o'clock I climbed into the Mustang and headed for the News Actuality studios.

The woman on the desk recognized me. The people in the elevator recognized me. I walked down the corridor and rang the bell next to the soundproof door with the numeric keypad.

Ricky Lee opened it. She was wearing a blue T-shirt and a short beige skirt. Her eyes were shining, the way they had shone last night, when I had thought it was the reflection of the sequins. She kissed me on the mouth, took my hand, and pulled me in. "Edward," she said. "Edward's the assistant editor on the six o'clock hour. He's a good friend. This is George."

Edward was thin, with a studio-pale face, a shaved head and red windowpane glasses. He said, "Glad to meet you. Have a seat."

I sat down on one of the swivel chairs in front of the editing board. "Center screen," said Edward. "Ricky thought you'd like to see it all run together."

Ricky Lee squeezed my hand under the table. The screen flashed a couple of times. A globe of the Earth appeared, cracked open. Clips of world events spilled out. There was an anchorman. The anchorman started talking.

"That's the first one," said Ricky Lee.

I recognized it. There was the story of Bill's death, the wreck of *Auk/PloughShare*. Then there was Rhyd with a string section, playing "The Alleluia Tree." Then there was me, looking haggard and disorientated under the TV lights, telling the story of what I had seen in Ethiopia, and Poliakoff posing against sacks of aid corn. It seemed a very long time ago. But it still looked to me like a masterly bit of television, combining maximum tear-jerking with furious narrative drive.

"Look at the next one," said Ricky Lee.

The next one had been done at my third jewels-and-skeletons luncheon. There were shots of the audience, then of me. I was less haggard, more confident. It had been skillfully cut. The humanitarian bits were still there, but this time they had used sentences from my speech that spoke of revenge and action. Where I had tried to balance anger and compassion, they had chosen anger. After the speech excerpts, there was film of the boys, much younger, that they must have prised out of Rhyd's record company; and a *vox pop* in the crowd, saying that whoever had done this to Walters and those kids should be caught and put away.

I could feel my hand becoming clammy in Ricky Lee's. The television was presenting the quotes so they said things I had not said. I was not surprised that Warren Diglis had thought violence was the only way of diverting me.

The next film had the same anchorman. It revolved around the Mrs. Senator Corin Johanssen lunch. "The Devis Crusade," said the anchorman. He outlined my progress to date, skated across the cause. He said, "The crusade continues." They had put the cameras low down under the lectern, catching the hands, so the little movements I made while I was talking looked odd and exaggerated. I was talking about the Alleluia Tree. There was no explanation of the Alleluia Tree or where it fitted. It came out of left field, in a low, Biblical whisper. It sounded like Oral Roberts on amphetamines.

My forehead was covered in cold sweat.

"Wait," said Ricky Lee.

They had Senator Johanssen on. "He is a real brave young man," said the Senator across his long New England jaw. "He is totally committed to his cause. He has attracted a lot of important donations, and I wish him every success."

The interviewer said, "Would you call him a fanatic?"

The Senator wagged his silver head. "You better believe it," he said.

Cut.

"We got some tape from today," said Edward.

"Go on," I said.

There was a good buildup: smiling faces, mob scenes, roars of applause. Then there was me, wild-eyed, shining with sweat. I had my arms out; they had been clapping, but there was no clapping on the tape. In a big, echoing hush, I said: "I am going to stop this man. Dead."

"Okay," said Edward. "They didn't assemble it yet."

Ricky Lee still had the sequins in her eyes. I said, "Bloody hell."

"Bloody hell why?"

"That's not what I said."

"It's what you mean, isn't it?" said Edward.

"They've taken it all out of context," I said.

"You mean it or you don't," said Edward. "That's the magic of television."

People kept using that phrase.

I was thinking about what Pierce had said to me in the car last night, on the way from the Shady Grove to the *Duchess of Malfi.* "Serge needs a feel-good factor. You're it."

Ricky Lee said, "You're meeting Hamil tomorrow, right? That's why I wanted you to see that. So you'll be careful."

I squeezed her hand. "I'll be careful," I said. I was thinking: How much of this will this Hamil have seen?

Ricky Lee said, "Are you staying in Portsmouth?"

"Yes." I was looking at the sequins in her eyes, but I was thinking: You are meeting Hamil tomorrow. Hamil is the man who killed Camilla, who is the cause of Joe and Harry's suffering. Like Edward the editor said: You mean it or you don't.

I meant it, all right.

I said, "Why don't you come along?"

33

W E PICKED UP SCOTCH JOHN FROM RECEPTION AND HEADED north. In the car, John said, "Good day?"

I told him it had been.

"Me too," he said. "I went visiting Warren Diglis."

I jerked my head around. The Mustang swerved. He was sitting crosswise in the small back seat, fiddling with a piece of string. I said, "Why?"

He said, "His boy Gerard give me one bad headache. I thought I would maybe sue him, common assault, you know?"

I said, "You're crazy."

He grinned at me. I noticed that inside the beard his lip was split. "I guess so," he said.

"So what happened?"

"His boy Gerard punched me out," said John. "Then he threw me down the steps."

"Another headache," I said.

"Making two," said John. "But I laid one of 'em out first." He sounded as if it might have been worthwhile. "Oh," he said. "He gave me something for you." He passed me an envelope.

I slit it with my thumb, glancing between it and the road. It was a sheet of cheap red paper, folded, covered in large black print. I pulled over, gave the wheel to Ricky Lee and went and sat in the passenger seat.

It was a campaign leaflet for Ras Hamil. It was in an English that must have been translated from Amharic, probably for circulation in Warren Diglis's pro-Hamil pressure group. At the top was a smudged black-and-white photograph of a thin Ethiopian man in military uniform. He could have been the colonel I had met in the office where the whitewash flakes trembled in the electric fan, except that he had a broken nose, and he was smiling. Under the photograph was a list. It said:

> NO to corruption
> YES to local power
> NO to World Bank big projects
> YES to village initiatives
> NO to multinational colonialism
> YES to local control

It went on like that.

I found I was getting angry. It was seductive stuff all right. It was a list of the planks in the platform Rhyd and Camilla had supported. Hamil had stolen it wholesale to make himself look good to his supporters overseas, while he—the anticorruption candidate opposed to interference from abroad—was running his campaign on the proceeds of corruption and murdering anyone who got in his way.

I crumpled the paper and shoved it in my pocket. Ricky Lee was looking across at me. "You okay?" she said.

"Fine," I said. I was fine. I was greatly looking forward to meeting the author of the manifesto and going through it point by point.

Ricky Lee took my hand in hers. "Take it easy," she said.

The pressure of her hand gave me other things to think about. I grinned at her, to show her everything was fine.

Poliakoff Communications had booked us into the Portsmouth, New Hampshire, Adler, a Poliakoff Hospitality Group Hotel, thirty-odd miles north of Boston, handy for the National Dynamics factory. The hall porter was covered in buttons. He said, "Saw you on the news tonight, Mr. Devis." John looked at me, Ricky Lee, and the Niagara Falls chandelier in the lobby. He muttered something in his beard about a drink, grabbed his room key, and vanished into the night.

"Portsmouth, Sunday, eleven o'clock," said the hall porter, hefting our trifling bags. "He'll be lucky."

Ricky Lee squeezed my hands and looked at me sideways out of her Irish-Chinese eyes. A bellboy showed us to a room, accepted ten dollars and reversed out. Ricky Lee sat down on the bed. "I can think of things you can do in Portsmouth on a Sunday at eleven o'clock," she said.

She turned the light out. The glass wall of the room filled with the moon and the shift of city lights in the black water of the harbor. Her clothes had gone. Her body was ivory in the moonlight, but warm when I took her in my arms. It was just as well to be warm, two people in a room with a glass wall, locked together under the moon. Tomorrow was not going to be anything like this. Stay warm while you can.

A lot later, Ricky Lee said, "I love you."

I moved my mouth an inch, so my lips were touching her ear. I said, "Snap."

"You poets," she said, and went to sleep.

Next thing I knew, the room was full of ice-gray light. Outside the window was white cotton wool, faintly tinged with orange. As I watched, a red-hot ball floated over a white bank, vanished. Ricky Lee's hair was a reddish tangle beside me on the pillow, her body a long mound under the bedclothes. I swung my feet out of bed, shoveled coffee into the coffee maker. Last night was leaving me. My stomach was knotted tight.

The smell of coffee woke her. She opened an eye. She said, "I still love you."

"Still snap."

She looked at me with her odd greenish eyes. She said, "What's on your mind?"

I smiled, a smile that did not feel even fifty percent genuine. I said, "Nothing."

She said, "Your sister?"

I did not have enough saliva to explain. I said, "I don't like heights." Then I rolled out of bed and into the shower.

Room service brought breakfast. We ate in silence, watching the white wads of fog rolling across the harbor. Scotch John met us in reception. Nice little convention at the Portsmouth Adler: dope dealer, folksinger, prophet of doom. We walked out into the cold gray car park.

Ricky Lee said, "Do airships fly in fog?"

I had been wondering. I slammed the car door and turned on the six o'clock weather.

"Fog," said the voice. "Winds southwesterly, ten to twenty, pushing a lot of warm air across a lot of cold sea. It could clear in places, but don't count on it. Weak front heading slowly south."

The fog was thick enough to condense on the windscreen. We drove across the river, then turned right past a gray shoal of warships in the Naval Shipyard, following the directions on Marlene's sheet of paper, peering through the windscreen wipers. After a couple of miles, the road ran alongside a chainlink fence topped with a coil of razor wire. Inside the fence was a flat green area of what might have been reclaimed marsh. Two huge buildings loomed indistinctly in the fog. Hangars. And another shape.

"There it is," said Ricky Lee.

My mouth felt as if it was full of corn dust again. The other shape was beyond the hangars: a fat gray cigar, floating horizontal ten feet above the ground, with a cabin slung under its belly. I did not grasp its size until something underneath it moved. The thing underneath it was a five-ton truck, but it looked the size of an ant.

None of us was saying anything now.

A sign on the fence said NATIONAL DYNAMICS—HOME OF A NEW GENERATION OF DIRIGIBLES. There was a gate with a gatehouse and a jeep parked outside. I showed my pass to a security man. He touched the peak of his cap in a semimilitary salute. He said, "Welcome to the base, Mr. Devis. Would you please follow Daryl here?"

His colleague walked to a gray jeep, raised an arm, and drove down a straight black road lined with whitewashed boulders. Gulls hung in the fog above the gray-green sward on either side. We drove to a range of long, low buildings between the giant hangars. Daryl climbed down from the jeep and said, "Maybe you would step this way, sir?" He opened a door in the side of the building. I climbed a couple of steps and went in.

A black man was waiting. He was wearing a dark gray business suit with a tie bearing a device made of the interlocked letters ND. He said, "Good morning, Mr. Devis. I'm Ralegh Harrison, as in Sir Walter. I've been asked to brief you on your forthcoming flight."

I said, "Will we fly in fog?"

Harrison smiled, his white teeth flashing under the fluorescent strip light in the office. "Sure will," he said. "One of the many plus points of the dirigible. Total control. You can take off and land at nil ground speed, get above that stuff. Then you go where you like." He opened a desk drawer and pulled out a flat black box the size of a romantic novel. "Here you are," he said. "Digital audiotape. Broadcast quality." He frowned at my jacket. "We have a holster. You can wear it under your shirt. Coat off, please. Unbutton. Arms up."

I raised my arms. He strapped the recorder to my left side. The holster was padded, so it was comfortable to wear.

"Okay," he said, fiddling with my jacket. "We've given you a special display handkerchief. Broadcast-quality mike in there." He grinned. "Automatic level control. No problem with background noise. You've got one-touch recording. Switch in the left-hand pocket. There's no playback. We'll do that for you when you get down. Put the coat on again."

I put it on.

"Undetectable in everyday wear," said Harrison. "As used by the FBI. Sit with your left side to the interviewee, close as you can."

Through the window I could see John and Ricky Lee waiting in the car. Ricky Lee was staring at us, her face still and solemn. Harrison said, "Other party not due for a little while yet." He pulled my jacket straight, stepped back in the manner of a tailor. "Real smart," he said. "Now if you'd sign this release?"

The piece of paper absolved Poliakoff Industries of all liability for any claims I might make. I signed.

The security man who had led us from the gatehouse came in. Harrison said, "Show Mr. Devis around the hangar. Give him the grand tour." He smiled. "Y'all have a nice flight, now!"

I shook him by the hand and forced a grin through a face stiffened with apprehension. I said, "You don't mind if my friends come too?"

His smile flickered. "I have no instructions on this," he said.

I said, "I presume Mr. Ras Hamil is going to have his . . . escort. I'd like to bring mine."

He frowned. He said, "Excuse me." He went into another office. I could hear the murmur of his voice through the wall. He came back, lips pursed, looking grave. He said, "I'm afraid that's not possible. Passholders only to fly. Mr. Poliakoff's personal stipulation." He cleared his throat. "Mr. Hamil will be flying with a single bodyguard. The airship crew have been briefed. I have been instructed to point out that the bodyguard was a condition or stipulation for Mr. Hamil's agreeing to the flight. Naturally, Mr. Hamil and his escort will be skin-searched before boarding."

I thought: Nothing can happen on an airship. I had Serge Poliakoff's personal assurance.

Daryl went outside and spoke to John and Ricky Lee. I watched through the window. Behind the misty windscreen, Ricky Lee's face was pale and set, as if she was worrying. I was nervous and excited, the way I had been on *Auk/PloughShare* in

309

Plymouth, before the start of the race. Not looking forward to it, but impatient for the start. As usual, it was hard to tell what was going on in John's mind. Daryl returned and took me on a tour of the offices.

There were people sitting in front of computers. None of them looked up. "Gasbag above," said Daryl, waving at a plan on a screen. "Helium, with ballonets. Pump air in and out of the ballonets, increase or decrease the weight of the ship. You go up and down according. Gondola, divided in two. Pilot and copilot in their own cabin. Then a passenger gondola, minimum weight, built of Kevlar and epoxy. Bulletproof, sound resistant. Nice steady working platform. Designed for anti-submarine work. But that's going out of style, so we're pushing it for mineral prospecting, aerial photography, military surveillance."

I nodded. It was the Poliakoff sales pitch. I was sweating under the recorder harness. Outside the window, the silvery gray gasbag shifted in the fog like a nervous whale. I wanted to get it over with.

"Ever been up before?" said Daryl cheerfully.

I shook my head. I did not trust myself to speak.

"You'll love it," said Daryl. "Let's take a drive around."

We walked out to the jeep. It was a longer drive than I had expected. The dirigible hung over us, big as a thundercloud. It was moored by the nose to a mast on the bed of a heavy four-wheel-drive truck and anchored to the ground by guywires. It shifted gently, like a boat anchored in a weak tide. A dozen men in white overalls were standing around the truck. They were big, and they looked fit. "Ground crew," said Daryl. He drove slowly down the length of the airship, talking. "One hundred and eighty feet long," he said. He pointed upward, at two hefty Terylene ropes running back from the nose to a pair of tobogganlike skids on the bottom of the gondola. "Mooring and launching lines." There were other wires, running back from the gondola to the rudder and ailerons standing out from the pointed back end of the gasbag like the fins of a bomb. "Control wires." On either side of the gondola was a six-foot airfoil strut, with an aero engine on the end. "Whole thing's an airfoil," said Daryl. "Captain'll fly you off like a heavier-than-air plane. Use a little fuel, lighten up. Then you're a power-assisted balloon. Like an auxiliary sailing ship, right?"

I said, "What if the engines stop?"

He grinned his enthusiast's grin. "They won't stop. And if they do, you're a balloon. Floating. Not like wings. You have water ballast. Dump it and you can stay up there for ever, like a ship, drifting." He looked across. "Hey," he said. "You nervous?"

I smiled. It felt like a facial cramp. "No," I said. I could hardly think about Ras Hamil. It was the idea of flying that was getting to me.

There were two men sitting in the forward compartment of the gondola. One of them was reading aloud from what might have been a manual. The other was setting switches and dials above the windscreen.

"Great," said Daryl. "Just enjoy yourself."

A stretch Lincoln with black windows had glided around the corner of the hangar. New sweat broke in my palms.

"It's the other guys," said Daryl. "I guess we should go say hello."

I said, dry-mouthed, "I'll meet them aboard."

Daryl shrugged. "Sure," he said.

The limousine's doors opened. Three men got out. One of them was Serge Poliakoff. The other two were tall, dressed in khaki overcoats. They were both black. The one in front was Ras Hamil. The other one was nearly seven feet tall. He would be a bodyguard.

Suddenly the flying was not the most daunting part of the day.

I opened the jeep door and jumped out. The air was cool and wet on my face. The tape machine chafed against the sweaty skin over my ribs. I shoved my hands into my pockets to stop them shaking and walked under the belly of the airship.

Poliakoff was talking. I saw his eyes flash at me. He made a quick gesture of his hand, which might have been to emphasize something he was saying, but involved a pointing movement at the airship.

"If you'd like to step aboard, sir?" said a voice.

There was another man in a white overall with NATIONAL DYNAMICS in Day-Glo print across the shoulders. He was standing by the foot of a ladder that bridged the four feet between the gondola and the ground. I swallowed hard, nodded. Poliakoff and the two black men were walking toward the airship. Poliakoff waved. I waved back. I went up the ladder.

It was like an airplane cabin. There were eight seats, arranged in pairs on either side of a central aisle. At the front end of the aisle was a door in a partition between the passenger department and the pilot's cabin. The man in the overall said, "Right at the back, please."

I said, "Please seat Mr. Hamil beside me."

The man in the white overall said, "That's all arranged, Mr. Devis. Welcome aboard."

I went and sat at the back on the right-hand side, so the microphone was next to the aisle, as per Ralegh Harrison's instructions. Under my window a couple of ground crew were taking neat little sandbags out of a locker in the gondola's side. The pilot turned his head at me, raised a hand. He had a big brown moustache and yellow fog glasses. He looked confident. I was reassured.

There was a smell of polyester resin and gasoline. It took me back to the Cessna, the day this man Ras Hamil had killed Rhyd and Camilla. The airship shifted at its mooring. Overhead in the gasbag, machinery whirred. It sounded like a pump. Ballonets, I thought. Pump the air in, pump the air out. Outside, Poliakoff's voice cried, "All aboard!"

Feet clattered on the ladder. A head appeared in the doorway. It was black, with curly hair, hair that grew straight out for perhaps four inches, in a halo. The forehead was high. The nose had once been narrow and aquiline, but someone or something had smashed it into a crooked S. The skin was cratered with pockmarks; the eyes were dark brown, fierce, with a yellow tinge to the whites.

CLAWHAMMER

I knew the face from the election leaflet. I was back where I had started, in the village, with the smell of ashes in my nostrils and the sun like a hot anvil on my skull.

"At the back, please, Colonel Hamil," said the voice of the ground crew charge hand. "On the left, if you would be so kind."

Hamil walked toward me, stooping. He was very tall and thin. He nodded at me, coiled himself into the seat. "So," he said. "We take a trip around the bay." His English was English English, with only the faintest of accents. He smiled. It was a huge, white smile.

Smile on, you bastard, I thought. You killed my sister. You will not be smiling for long.

Something caught my eye outside the window. It was Ricky Lee, standing on the concrete apron, waving. I waved back. Then I realized that she was beckoning me toward the ladder.

I got up, moving awkwardly to conceal the recorder strapped to my ribs. I stuck my head out of the door.

She said, "Kiss me goodbye."

I went down the ladder. A man in white overalls was taking sandbags out of a compartment. Poliakoff was standing on one side, grinning a God-bless-you-my-children grin.

Ricky Lee pulled my face down to hers. "That guy," she said. "The black guy in the office. What was he all about?"

"He gave me a tape recorder."

She said, "He was at the Birdman elevator with Jackson and Gerard. He drove their car."

"Seats please," said the pilot over a Tannoy.

"All aboard," said Poliakoff, jolly as the captain of the *Skylark*. He was looking at his watch. "Tight schedule here."

I was halfway up the ladder. I did not understand. Things were happening too quickly. Something was wrong.

I shuffled down the gangway, sat down in my seat.

The pilot pulled on a pair of earphones. The Tannoy crackled. "Good morning, gentlemen," it said. "Please fasten your seat belts. We're going for a quick takeoff here. We have a little window in the fog, and I believe that there are some press gentlemen we should get out of the way of." There was a rising howl left and right as the engines started.

The men in white overalls had unlashed the big mooring lines from the gondola skids. They were holding them taut like tent guyropes, triangulating the downward pull under the nose, six a side. A thirteenth man was up the mooring tower. He raised his hand. The nose floated free, uncoupled from the mast. The heavies in white overalls took the strain. Slowly, they walked us sideways, away from the mooring tower and out on to the grass of the field. The perspex window was like a TV screen. It would all have been unreal, except that the airship felt buoyant now, straining for the gray sky. Oh, Christ, I was saying at the back of my mind. We are going flying.

In the front of my mind was a puzzle as intractable as a crossword clue. If the man in the office worked for Warren Diglis, what was he doing harnessing me up with tape recorders for the benefit of Serge Poliakoff?

The men in white overalls had stopped walking. The pilot was flicking switches above his head.

The answer dawned on me suddenly, like the answer to a crossword clue. It made my heart ring like a hammer on an anvil.

Harrison did work for Poliakoff.

The engines roared up to full power. The men in white overalls let go the lines. The airship accelerated down the runway, bounced twice, and wallowed into the gray air.

34

*T*HE GONDOLA WAS TILTED UP AT A HORRIBLE ANGLE. THE COPILOT looked around at me. His face was blank, without curiosity. He turned his head away again, into the gray cotton wool streaming past the windscreen.

The pilot throttled back. The howl of the engines died to a snarl. Beyond the blunt nose of the airship the fog shredded and thinned. The huge cigar jumped out of the blanket of gray cotton wool and into the dazzling sunshine.

I could feel the straps of the tape recorder. Ras Hamil was staring at me, his smashed-up aristocrat's face creased with polite curiosity. He said, "Is everything all right?"

I said, "Fine."

Ras Hamil said, "I believe I am right in thinking that you are Camilla's brother?"

I stared at him. I could feel a cool breeze playing in my mouth.

"She did not tell you we knew each other?" said Ras Hamil.

I tried to tell him that she could not tell anyone anything, because he had killed her. What came out was a sort of croak. His eyes were resting upon me with the polite distress of a host at a tea party learning that cucumber sandwiches do not agree with one of his guests. "It was not a thing generally known," he said. "But Rhydian and Camilla were very good friends to me."

My voice was back, just. I said, "Is that why you killed them?"

He frowned. He said, "What makes you think that?"

My head was full of sun like hot anvils, and the bitter smell of ashes. I said, "I was told, by people I trust."

His eyebrows went up. He said, "You have been most gravely misled." His eyes had become remote, as if he was solving a problem in another compartment of his mind. "Rhydian and Camilla were among my most trusted advisers. I have known them . . . oh, years. Since they first came to Africa. It was Rhydian who first introduced me to the notions of permaculture. Did he not tell you?"

I shook my head. This man was telling me he could turn the world upside down.

And I was beginning to believe him.

"They were both my very dear friends. It was Camilla who helped me write my manifesto. Multinational colonialism. Does it not have that ring?"

I pulled from my pocket the red flyer Diglis had given Scotch John. My fingers felt big and stiff as cucumbers.

"She and Rhyd and the boys," said Hamil. "Many a time we have sat in the house by the Alleluia Tree." He reached into the breast pocket of his loose overcoat. My head was spinning. The man next to me should have been a warlord. Camilla and Rhyd should have been beneath his notice, two more corpses in the trail that marked his path.

But he knew them by name, and the boys. He knew about the Alleluia Tree. I did not want to believe him.

"Look," he said.

His hand was coming out of his overcoat. The gun, I thought. The knife. Attack, screamed a part of my mind. Get him before he gets you.

But I did not move.

The hand came out again. It was a long hand, slim fingered. It held a photograph taped to a piece of board, the tape yellow with age and much handling.

There were four people in the photograph. There were Rhyd and Camilla; Rhyd grinning, Camilla laughing, her blond ponytail hanging over the back of her homemade deckchair. The object of their amusement was Ras Hamil, who seemed to be telling a story, long hands molding the air in front of him, eyes bugged, eyebrows up by his hairline.

The fourth person was black. He was wearing a dun-colored uniform. He had a high, domed forehead and hair that sat on the back of his head like a yarmulke. He was smiling, but it was the smile of someone not quite at ease, who wanted to look as if he was part of things while keeping his distance.

The fourth person's name was Mr. Gugsa. I had met him under the burned-out limbs of the Alleluia Tree. He had said: *It is Ras Hamil who has done this thing.* Then I had run away.

My eyes were locked on Camilla's. Camilla, who did not know how to lie. Who was telling me something across the darkness that separated us. *Trust this man.*

I found I was shaking.

Poliakoff had told me things, too. He had put me on TV. Edward the editor had said: *You mean it or you don't. That's the magic of television.*

That was not the magic of television. The magic of television was that Serge Poliakoff could put George Devis on a screen and make him seem a crusader and a fanatic. Edit George Devis's speech at the Hunger Brunch, so all he seemed to have said was he was going to stop Ras Hamil, dead. Slowly and carefully, over a period of weeks, set George Devis up.

I remembered Poliakoff looking at his watch. Checking that we were running to timetable.

The airship of fools.

Ralegh Harrison was the dispatcher. The copilot was the supervisor. George Devis was the man who to get his revenge on the murderer of his sister and brother-in-law would stop at nothing.

Including his own death.

Saw the guy on TV, they would say. Weird, huh? Like, *crazy*. You could see that one coming all right, eh?

Below, a yellowish beach showed through a gray swirl of fog. I heard Rhyd's tape again: *Die with Mr. Coffee in the sand.*

Not coffee, as in breakfast.

Koffee, as in Poliakoff.

Poliakoff, the multinational colonialist. In whose interest it was to find extra markets for the produce of his factories.

Ras Hamil, committed to keeping people like Poliakoff out.

So Poliakoff had sent George Devis up into the sky with Ras Hamil in a bulletproof box. With a tape recorder strapped to him. Or something that looked like a tape recorder.

I felt as if the deck of the airship had turned to quicksand, like the corn in the bins at Birdman's. I was pouring sweat.

Sit with your left side to the interviewee, close as you can.

I pulled off my jacket, ripped my shirt open. The microphone wire tangled in the coat. I bundled the whole lot up together. The copilot was looking around again. His eyes met mine. He pulled back his fist and hit the pilot on the side of the head. The pilot flinched away. The copilot wound the big mahogany-bound wheel by his left hand. The horizon soared up the windscreen. The deck went from under my feet. I clung on to a seat leg, yanked open the gondola door. The howl of the engines filled the cabin. I flung the coat and tape recorder out as far as I could. They hung in the air, seeming to float toward the layer of fog, the sleeves of the coat flapping like vestigial wings, flying it forward along the side of the gondola past the pilot's side window.

There was a white flash and a clap of thunder that flung me back across the gondola and into the far wall. The air was full of the stink of burning. I landed on a seat, facing the partition that separated the passengers from the pilot. Ten seconds ago, the partition had been clear. Now it was streaked with red. My ears were ringing.

There was a clear patch remaining in the partition. Through

it, I could see that the pilot was no longer looking straight ahead. He was slumped sideways in his seat. The copilot had disappeared.

The nose climbed and climbed. There was a dreadful feeling of weightlessness. It began to sink again, too far. The airship wallowed on its side. I slid across the floor. My legs were out of the door, in the howl of the engines. I grabbed the tubular alloy support of the seat. My mind was roaring *No* as I hung suspended above the emptiness. A voice was yelling. My voice.

The airship lurched suddenly in the other direction. I crashed in. The door slid shut. I clung to a seat base, sobbing for breath. The engines faded to a low hum. The horizon leveled across the pilot's window.

I pulled myself up and into a seat. Ras Hamil's bodyguard was standing in front of Ras Hamil. His teeth were bared, his eyes bulging. He had the look of a dog, leashed back but ready to jump.

I was thinking: *Passenger gondola, minimum weight, built of Kevlar and epoxy.* Bulletproof waistcoats are made of Kevlar. And nail-bomb-proof gondolas. I could feel the void a thickness of composite away. Nausea swilled in my gut.

Ras Hamil said, in his polite, cultured voice, "Excuse me, what is this?"

I dragged myself out of my pit of vertigo. I said, "Someone strapped a bomb to me." My voice was not working properly.

The bodyguard twitched and snarled. Hamil said something in Amharic and he subsided. "I must thank you, then," said Hamil. "It appears you have saved my life."

I sat down. I stared at his pockmarked face and his decent brown eyes, and tried not to vomit all over him.

The airship droned on, nose up, like a pike hanging in a pond. Equilibrium. A long way to port, something long and low and solid rose from the fog like a headland from a sea. Maine. Up in the cabin, the pilot was slumped sideways in his seat. There was no sign of the copilot. We were over the Atlantic. We would stay up here until we ran out of fuel and became a balloon, God knew how many feet in the air, God knew how many miles out over the Atlantic, with a twenty-knot sou'westerly breeze under our tail.

I said, "Do either of you know how to fly a plane?"

Ras Hamil shook his head.

I walked gingerly forward to the door leading to the pilot's cabin. It was locked. The blood on the screen was turning brown. There was no movement from the pilot's body. I still could not see the copilot.

The engines hummed drowsily. The only thing that moved was the horizon, sliding quietly up the windscreen.

At first, I could not think what that meant. Then I worked it out.

My mouth turned dry again, and my knees weakened. I walked quickly back down the aisle. The horizon rose gently, steadied.

Ras Hamil said, "What is it?"

I opened my mouth to answer. No sound came out. I was looking at him and the bodyguard; the way their shoulders bulked out their greatcoats, the length of their legs. I was shorter and thinner. I would be an easy twenty pounds lighter.

I cleared my throat. Grin. Does you good. Gets blood into the head. Stops you fainting. I said, "I'm going to have to get into the cockpit."

Hamil said, "But the door is locked."

I said, "There's another. Stay here. Right at the back."

Ras Hamil understood. He said something to his bodyguard. The bodyguard moved into the seat in which I had begun the flight. Without giving myself time to think, I took the two steps up the aisle, got a firm grip on the back of a seat, and slid back the gondola door.

The sound of the engines became a roar. There was wind out there. Perhaps twenty knots, I thought. Not a lot.

Then I looked down.

There was a skid below the gondola; one skid a side, like the runners of a toboggan. Below the skid was perhaps three thousand feet of absolutely nothing at all.

When you are scared of heights, you have dreams like that, and you wake up screaming. But this was not a dream, and I did not have the breath to scream.

My knees turned to liquid. My stomach curdled. I shut my eyes.

Behind the eyelids, I made a resolution. Don't look down. Look sideways.

I craned my neck out of the door and turned my head into the wind. I opened my eyes.

The side of the gondola stretched away forward, silvery composite and portholes. After the third porthole, the side was no longer smooth. It had once been made largely of Plexiglas. Now there was a ragged hole. From the hole there dangled a foot. The pilot's foot. Beyond the pilot's foot was blue sky and gray horizon. I jerked my eyes back to the gondola.

I was going nicely now. Limited horizons. Achievable plans. There was a wire rope along the gondola's side at the level of the doorsill, threaded through eyes at two-foot intervals. It looked as if it might be useful for hanging equipment on.

Or as a handrail.

I leaned out, found the wire, tugged it. It held firm. I turned around, knelt on the floor and wriggled my legs out over the sill. The vibration of the engines came up through my ribcage. Under the seats, I saw the big, polished black shoes of Hamil and his bodyguard.

My own feet met resistance: the bar of the skid. The slipstream battered at my trouser legs. Ounce by ounce, I transferred my weight to my feet. The skid was hard and rigid, with a slight bounce, the way a boat will bounce in a ripple that does not amount to actual waves. A little voice was gibbering in my head. Floating in a sea of air, it said. They don't call them airships for nothing. Ho, ho, said the little voice. Very amusing. All the way up here.

The little voice got my whole weight onto the skid and my left hand onto the wire. Then it became silent, because I had taken the strain with the hand and shuffled sideways, and got the right hand onto the wire. And instead of my eyes seeing seat frames and big, frightened black shoes, I was looking at smooth, silvery composite, three inches from my nose.

And absolutely nothing else.

My knee joints were locked. The howl of the engines tore at my ears. I shuffled a step, moved my clawed fingers along the wire, shuffled another step.

I got into a rhythm. Inch by inch, I thought. It was getting better. I felt light.

Light.

I glanced sideways. There was the silver plastic side and the pilot's leg dangling in the slipstream. After the leg, there was the horizon. The horizon was creeping upward. I froze. The skid was sinking like a quicksand. I saw a picture of myself: an ant-sized figure, clinging to the huge floating cigar as the nose went down, down, and the engines screwed us into the fog, and whatever was underneath the fog.

Move, I thought.

I unfroze. I leaned my weight back, out over the void, and took two steps. The steps brought me to the bottom of the ladder leading from the skid to the pilot's cabin. As I climbed the ladder, I could feel my weight slumping to the left. The airship was diving. My stomach became lighter than air. I reached the top.

35

*T*HE DOOR HAD ONCE BEEN PLEXIGLAS. NOW IT WAS A BIG, splintered hole, through which the pilot's foot was dangling. I was in a hot sweat now, knees knocking. I shoved the pilot's foot back in. It was quite limp, with a horrible weight to it.

I hooked it around something, found the door catch with my left hand. What was left of the door slid aft. I went up the last rung of the ladder, stepped across the pilot's legs. I was in.

I got into the little space between the seats and let my knees shake like road drills. Above and in front of me, the gasbag was the nose of an overweight torpedo. To my right, the copilot was slumped sideways. There was a bruise on his forehead. His dark glasses were bent and hanging off his face. He was breathing.

The pilot's head was back. His glasses had gone. His eyes were closed. His face was spider-webbed with blood. There was blood on his coat, too, oozing from a jagged rip in the sleeve, and his left leg was bleeding, dark blood, oozing through a dozen rents in his trouser leg. He was breathing, too.

The voice in my head had started up again. This is what

happens to a man when you set off a nail bomb ten feet and a thickness of Plexiglas away from him. The nail bomb that was strapped to your own personal ribcage, ten inches away from the personal ribcage of Mr. Ras Hamil.

The cabin stank of blood. My gorge rose. No time for being sick. There were dials on a dashboard. I recognized one of them as an altimeter. It was unwinding through a thousand feet, the big hand moving as fast as the second hand on a watch. *Get the controls*, I thought. I leaned over, found the buckle of the pilot's seat belt. I stood in the space between the seats and pulled at his arm. He slumped sideways into the gap. I unlatched the door. It opened into the passenger cabin. I said, "Get this man. He's hurt."

Hamil's bodyguard came forward, dragged the pilot back. I edged into the pilot's seat. My fingers fumbled at the straps.

Blood had sprayed all over the instruments. A clod of shrapnel had ripped in and upward. There was something on the roof of the gondola that might once have been a radio. Now it looked like a portion of multicolored vermicelli.

I swallowed bone-dry nothing. No help from that direction.

The horizon had returned to the center of the windscreen. The altimeter had stopped unwinding at nine hundred feet. There were pedals under my feet. Rudder pedals. There was a wheel under my right hand. The aileron wheel. I rolled it forward. The horizon climbed up the windscreen. I rolled it backward. The horizon drifted downward. I made it steady.

I unbolted the connecting door. I shouted, "In here!"

Hamil's bodyguard came forward. His eyes moved around the cabin. I pulled back on the wheel to counter the effects of his weight. On my left, through the blown out door, wind and noise bellowed in from the void. I saw the beads of sweat pop on his forehead. I pointed at the copilot and yelled, "Shut the door!" pointing back into the passenger cabin.

He nodded. He put his hands under the copilot's armpits, picked him up as if he were light as a cat, and went aft.

It was cold in the pilot's seat. The sweat was congealing on my body. I felt light-headed with the aftereffects of chemicals released by terror.

I had flown in light aircraft as a passenger. Now all I had to do was make use of the information I had gathered in that passenger seat to become an airship pilot before the airship ran out of fuel.

Easy.

I started on the gauges. In front of me were four vertical white stripes with red bars in them. They looked like old-fashioned mercury barometers, except that the mercury was red. Something to do with the gasbag, I guessed. On its left were an altimeter and an artificial horizon and a turn-and-bank indicator. On its right were a rate-of-climb indicator and an airspeed indicator. In the center was a compass. In front of the copilot's seat were the engine dials and gauges.

The nausea receded. I was beginning to feel almost at home. Very gently, I applied my right foot to the right rudder pedal.

The mooring lines hanging from the nose began to move gently across the horizon to the right. There was a long, straight edge of cloud ahead, moving left. I was not paying any attention to long, straight edges of cloud, because I was pleased. The seat under me bounced slightly. It was not like an airplane with wings that could fall off. We were buoyant, floating. All you have to do, I thought, is turn this around, and drive it back the way you have come. Our course was 047° magnetic. The reciprocal of 047° is 227°. Foot on pedal. Around we go.

The mooring lines kept up their sweep across the horizon, and the numbers on the compass kept flicking. At 180°, they slowed. The airship banked left, away from the direction of the turn. I was sweating again. The mooring lines were not moving any more. They were blowing sideways. The airspeed indicator was giving the same reading: forty knots. The mooring lines started moving again.

They were moving the wrong way, right to left.

The sweat was squirting off me now. The idiot voice was

back, giving advice. Airship, it was saying. There's a wind. What do you do in a boat, under engine, if you're stuck in the current, and you can't get head-to-wind?

More power. More rudder.

I booted the rudder hard over, raised my hand to the throttles on the instrument panel above the windscreen, carefully, because there were a lot of dangerous-looking knobs up there. DUMP WATER BALLAST, said five yellow ones. There was a red one, with a guard over it. The red one said DUMP HELIUM. The blood drained from my head at the thought of DUMP HELIUM. Gently, I pushed forward the left-hand throttle.

The engine note in my left ear rose to a howl. The airframe started to judder, and the horizon tilted to the left. The nose climbed toward the eye of the wind.

I kept my hand on the throttle. As the nose came into the wind, I eased back. For a moment, the great silver torpedo hung on 227°. Then it went too far and the wind caught it and it swung, and I was blipping violently at the port throttle to hold it, and the gondola was bucking like a bronco as I got it up into the wind again. But up in the wind the nose fell away to port, and I was at the throttle and rudder again.

It happened half a dozen times. By the end, I was shaking with fear, and I knew that without a lot of hours' training as an airship pilot I was never going to be able to make any progress to windward.

I sat there and watched the mooring lines swing across the horizon and tried to think. The fuel gauges read half-full, but I had no idea what the capacity would be or how many tanks there were.

What we needed was dry land.

There was a pocket by the copilot's seat. In the pocket were what looked like maps and a clear plastic plotter. There was a gas mask, too. Whoever was arranging George Devis's murder-suicide had told the copilot about gas, not nail bombs. Touching, the way they looked after their employees. I threw the gas mask out of the wrecked pilot's door. Then I went through the maps, steadying them against the flap of the slipstream. We had been airborne for an hour and ten minutes by my watch. Assuming a twenty-knot wind, and forty knots forward speed under engines, we would be somewhere about ten miles south of Muscongus Bay.

So I found a pencil, and started drawing shaky vectors: ten miles north, quarter of an hour. Lay off for twenty knots of wind, five miles. Work out course to steer. It was how you dead-reckoned a boat. It ought to work for an airship.

I waved an arm. This time it was Ras Hamil who came forward. He sat in the copilot's seat. I said, "We'll fly across the wind. Find land."

He nodded, looking nervously at the gray fog beneath the open door on my left. He said, "I shall owe you a great debt."

I said, "We're not there yet." The muscles on my face felt tight. I realized I was grinding my teeth. I throttled up, steered to port. The airframe juddered hard as the slipstream crossed the rudder. The nose began to come around the horizon. Hamil said something over the howl of the engine. I yelled, "What?"

The engine note flattened. Hamil said, "Your sister would have been very proud of her brother."

He had finished the sentence in complete silence. I was not paying him any attention.

I was looking at the fuel gauge. Its needle was suddenly below the zero, resting on the pin.

Hamil's bodyguard shouted something from the gondola. Hamil said, "He says it smells of gasoline."

I shoved the rudder control with my right foot. Nothing happened. I was sweating again. I knew why it could be smelling of gasoline.

Take a fuel line. Blow up a nail bomb ten feet away from it so a fitting gets a dent or a crack. Then throttle up your engines, both at once, and turn your airship into the wind so the whole thing judders like a Channel ferry in a heavy sea.

Bang goes the fitting. Bang goes the gasoline.

Hamil said, "What is this?"

I said, "I think we've run out of fuel."

"Ah." For all the worry on his face, I could have said that the weather was exceptionally clement for the time of year. "So we still fly?"

"If the engines stop, we're a balloon." I was quoting the ground crew. "We can stay up here forever."

"Good," said Hamil. His eyes rested on me, tranquil as agates. "Who told you I had killed your sister?"

I said, "Mr. Gugsa."

Hamil smiled. He took out his photograph again. He put a finger on the face of the man in the dun-colored uniform with the skullcap of hair. The finger paled with the pressure. "Mr. Gugsa," he said. "When I was a guerrilla, he fought with me. He is a good fighter, but a cruel man. When the fighting had finished, the talking began. We were all seeking a way that my poor country could make its way in the world. Battle is giving way to politics. But for many like Gugsa, talking is only desert breeze, wasted time. They missed the naked women begging for mercy in the huts, the strong feeling they got when they cut the manhood from the body of their enemy. So Gugsa left me. I had trusted him, fool that I was. When he left, he took with him some secrets that Rhydian and I had found out."

The airship had found a balance, nose up, drifting.

I said, "Such as the affair of Eugene Wollo and the corn."

He nodded. "Such as that affair," he said. "Truly, you nursed at the same breast as Camilla Walters."

I said, "I was told that the money raised by Wollo went to finance your political ambitions."

He laughed, a sharp guffaw, like the cough of a lion. "Not my political ambitions. The political ambitions of people who do not think as I do. Wollo gets his corn from people who want a government in my country that will buy the things they make in their factories. People like Gugsa work for Wollo because they want the kind of power that made them love war." He sighed. "Your sister and Rhyd Walters worked with their minds, stone from the ground, water from the sky, the seeds of plants. All these things occur naturally in my country. But people like Serge Poliakoff tell me that when I have power, I will be needing to buy an airship." He laughed again. "How useful an airship will be," he said, "in a country where camels are dying of thirst, which in a week or a year may not even be a country. Obviously we need an airship, the way a rhinoceros needs an embroidery frame." He waved a long hand in the air. "Mr. Poliakoff expects that if he puts money for me in Switzerland, I will one day buy this thing for more money than we spend on schools in a year." He frowned. "Or so he pretends. It seems, though, that he wants to kill me, and you too, in his airship."

I said, "But it was the U.S. government that was sending corn to Wollo."

"Not the U.S. government," he said.

"The Emergency Resources Bureau."

He shook his head. "The ERB is not a government organization. Rhydian has told me."

I stared at him. Charis Brown had told me the opposite. "Are you sure?"

He sighed. "I think that this is the reason he is dead," he said. "He said that this ERB is set up like a private organization, but those who run it let it be known to anyone who is interested that it is a front organization for the commercial branch of the CIA. We believe it is owned by a company that thinks it has found big minerals in the Red Sea. Metalliferous nodules. Also perhaps oil. They were channeling corn as a form of payment, to support the parties in Ethiopia that have been corrupted by the . . . multinational colonialists. I know that your sister and Rhydian were getting close to these people and the source of their funds. The ERB found their life was getting difficult; they were attracting attention, they could not tell how. So they marked a consignment of corn in some way, to find out who was collecting evidence against them. I believe that is how they tracked Rhyd."

I stared at him. Bill had brought back a sample of the corn Rhyd had tracked down as an exhibit in the case against the ERB, not in the case against Ras Hamil.

Lucky for Poliakoff he had died.

And lucky for Poliakoff that George Devis the poet had been

so eager to expiate his cowardice and avenge his sister that he had charged in, fists flailing, eyes shut, mouth open, so Poliakoff could feed him the whole thing upside down. I had swallowed it. And now Ras Hamil and I were meant to be dead in a nice, newsworthy murder-suicide. And in Ethiopia the field would be clear for Poliakoff, who knew that mineral rights were what you needed in life, and that dreamers were dangerous, unless you could feed into their dreams monsters that turned out to be real.

But I knew who the monsters were, now. And they had failed to kill us.

So it was our turn.

Hamil said, "I wish to go down to the ground, to tell people what has happened to us." He frowned. "But I suppose that without evidence, we may not be believed."

I said, "There is evidence."

Hamil said, "I had believed it burnt in the house in the village."

"I don't think so." The airship felt light and purposeless, like a drifting boat. Hundreds of feet below, the fog was a sheet of dull pearl. To the north, the line of cloud was much closer.

It was a long line of cloud, its ends out of sight over the horizon. A weak front, heading slowly south. The weatherman had described it. The rim of a lump of cool air, meeting the warm southern air that was causing the fog.

It had possibilities, this front.

I told Hamil what I was going to try to do. His smile did not falter. At the end he went aft, to talk to his bodyguard.

There were four little switches below the dials in front of me, the ones that looked like mercury barometers without the mercury. They were marked FORE, AFT, MIDSHIPS and ALL. My mind was dredging around in the children's encyclopedia that had festered on a shelf in the dark passage of the vicarage when I had been perhaps eight. The article had been headed "The Wondrous Zeppelin." There had been pictures of a cathedral-sized interior, scaffolded with aluminum girders and bloated with doped silk hydrogen bags. The National Dynamics airship was kept aloft with helium, not hydrogen, but that was not important. The important thing was that in the gasbags had been other bags called ballonets. The ground crew had mentioned ballonets. By pumping air in and out of these bags, raising and lowering its pressure, you could regulate the weight of the airship. Make it lighter, it rose. Make it heavier, it fell.

Just now the sun was shining on the gasbag, causing the helium to expand, and we had risen to fourteen hundred feet.

I swallowed. I leaned forward, and gingerly twisted the button marked ALL to the left.

Somewhere above me in the gasbag, motors whined. My heart began thumping hard. I kept my eyes on the altimeter.

Very slowly, the minute hand began to unwind. We dropped a hundred feet. The rate-of-climb indicator said we were going down at five feet a second. Well done, I thought.

The airship was turning gently about its own axis now. The edge of the cloud was much closer. It was a long gray cliff, stretching northwest/southeast across the sky as far as the eye could see. When I craned my neck up, the sky above the curved flank of the gasbag looked hazy with little feathers of cirrus.

I sat there and waited, wiping my palms on my jeans.

The cloud covered the sky. The sun went out as if someone had turned off a light. The gondola began to buck and shudder as the gasbag hit flaws in the stronger wind under the cloud. The air coming through the wrecked pilot-side door was suddenly much colder. Below, something was happening to the roof of fog over the world. One moment it was writhing up in great plumes like the sun's mantle in an eclipse. The next, it was gone.

In its place was sea the color of tarmac. We were low enough to see the white horses chasing each other diagonally toward a sprawl of islands to the northwest.

It is one thing making a careful plan. It is another to be

sitting in a fifty-five-meter airship you do not know how to fly, being blown toward the plan's fruition at better than twenty knots. I felt sick. The moisture that should have been in my mouth was on my hands.

I watched out of the windscreen. The gray and black map of islands and sea inched by to the left. Under a front, you sometimes get a sudden kink in the isobars, a shift of wind. It should shove us over the land.

This time, there seemed to be no shift of wind.

Disappointment settled in my stomach like a block of lead. The gondola bounced and swayed.

It was hard to tell exactly where we were heading, because the airship was spinning, end past end, embedded in the lump of cold air heading northeast. The islands filed past, backed by the heavier, blacker mass of the mainland.

After ten minutes, there seemed to be something black up ahead: a long, low shape, buried in the sea. The wind blew. It came close. It was land. Islands. If we had been facing in the direction we were traveling, it would have been possible to describe it as fine on the port bow.

I reached out for the knob that said ALL, twisted it left. Up in the envelope, the servos whined. The altimeter unwound: nine hundred feet, eight hundred, down through six hundred, four hundred. The whitecaps were much closer now. We were passing over them at frightening speed.

The wind blows in a different direction at the masthead than on the deck. The higher you are, the harder it blows. So the lower you are, the softer it blows. And the softer it blows, the freer it blows.

I pumped air into the ballonets in tentative sips until the altimeter showed a hundred feet. The sound of the sea was a dull hiss and roar in the door now, and over the stench of the pilot's blood came the tang of salt. The islands on the horizon were coming closer. They looked like a crocodile with its neck under water, head facing out to sea. As far as I could tell, down here almost at sea level, we were making a course for its shoulder blades. I pawed at the map with fingers that did not want to cooperate. The crocodile's back was Matinicus Island, with Ragged Island to seaward.

I shouted, "Coming up."

There was no need to shout, but there seemed to be a lot of static in my mind. I saw out of the corner of my eye Hamil and the bodyguard laying the bodies of the unconscious pilot and copilot close to the gondola door. There was the rumble and click of the door opening. I shouted, "Wait for it!"

The island was an island now, low and flat, stretching across the nose; black woods, fields gray-green in the dull light filtering through the cloud base. My fingers caressed the ALL button. The altimeter read eighty feet, sinking. A lobster boat passed below. There were two faces, looking up. One of them was wearing dark glasses. We were too low. I twisted the button again, yanked one of the yellow DUMP WATER knobs. A white beach appeared at the foot of a foreshore of pines. We were rising again. Miss the pines, I thought. The beach slid out of the field of view as the airship spun. I was looking at gray sea and white horses. The beach came back, underneath us now. A treetop whipped by ten feet from my left foot. There was grass, traveling at twenty knots, then a belt of trees. Beyond the trees was what might have been a meadow. We were moving toward it right side forward. For the door to be usable, we need to be left side forward. I was running out of good ideas. I found the FORE ballonet button, twisted it. Pumps whined. I shouted, "Hold on!" The nose dipped toward the trees, slow and graceful as an elephant's trunk. I thought: This is a bad idea.

It hit.

There was a crash of branches that filled the cabin. The airship began to slew. We were sixty yards long, traveling at twenty-five knots. The slew turned into a sort of diagonal-axis cartwheel, the tail sweeping up and over, flicking downwind as the mooring lines on the nose snagged in the last of the trees. The airship gave a huge, ponderous wriggle and lay head-to-wind, fifty feet above the ground. I twisted the ALL button. It sank. The skids hit the ground with a bang. I shouted, "Jump!" and climbed out of the seat.

Back in the gondola, Hamil had the pilot under the armpits,

passing him through the door down to the bodyguard. The copilot was lying in the gangway, where he had slithered when the airship had cartwheeled.

The deck lurched under my feet. Forward, the mooring ropes were writhing like snakes in the trees. Someone was shouting. We were slipping back downwind.

Hamil let the pilot go, jumped himself. I started back down the aisle.

Relieved of Hamil's weight, the airship bounced thirty feet into the air. A gust of wind bowed the crests of the pine trees. It lurched again, leaped upward, rolled on to its right side, the one that made it impossible to use the door, even if the door had not been a hundred feet off the ground. I fell, skidded down the aisle of the gondola, tripped over the copilot. There was a series of bangs, each one as loud as a car crash. I was lying on a window, looking down at a green meadow. On the meadow were a flock of miniature sheep, and two black faces with white eyeballs, and a crumpled figure lying between them.

Then the faces were too small for me to see the eyeballs any more. Then there was no meadow. I crawled into the cockpit. There was the altimeter, reading 120 feet and climbing, and below the windows the blacktop sea.

36

*T*HE HORIZON SPUN PAST THE WINDSCREEN: SEA, ISLAND, SEA, SEA. Next time it spun, I could see both ends of the island at the same time. The time after that, I could see the far side of the island, and the island itself like a green map, the meadow in the trees the size of a pocket handkerchief.

The altimeter read 1100 feet. The turbulence was less up here. I crept with shaky knees to the pilot's seat and buckled myself in.

Ras Hamil was on the ground, in possession of Ricky Lee's telephone number and an array of facts incriminating to Serge Poliakoff. I was in the air, in possession of an airship and an unconscious copilot, with a steady breeze shoving us in the general direction of Greenland. There were consolations. There would be helicopters out. And when the helicopters found us, the copilot would have things to tell us. Like what his exact instructions had been, and whom they had come from.

The altimeter hit two thousand feet. We were just below the gray roof of cloud. It was smooth up here, without bumps. I was getting handy with the ballonet controls. I established a height, stabilized, and walked aft into the passenger cabin.

The copilot was lying on his back. He was breathing easily. His eyes were closed. So was his mouth. He had a thick neck, close-cropped black hair, blue-shadowed jowls. He looked more like an infantryman than a pilot. One of Poliakoff's foot soldiers. I rolled him on to his side into the recovery position. In the back of my mind, I was thinking: Something is wrong. But I could not work out what.

Right at the back, between the seat, was a red arrow. Below the arrow, stenciled letters said LIFE RAFT—10 PERSONS. I pulled the hatch off. The life raft was in a canister, all present and correct. That was a consolation, anyway.

The feeling in the back of my mind faded. For a moment, I had the idea that things were going well.

Only for a moment.

In the corner of my vision, something flickered. I half turned. I had time to get my left hand halfway up to ward off whatever was going to happen. Something hit me very hard on the muscle of the upper arm. My hand was numb. I was looking into the face of the copilot. His skin was greenish-gray. His mouth was open now. The thought in the back of my mind rushed to the front, too late. Unconscious men's mouths are open, not shut. He had been faking.

There was a fire extinguisher in his right hand. The fire extinguisher he had hit me with. I tried to hit him with my right hand. My knuckles hit ribs. My left hand was not working.

His fingers were fumbling with the extinguisher. Trying to get the safety pin out. He might have been feigning unconsciousness, but he was concussed all right. I pulled my foot back to smash him in the kneecap.

He jerked his head forward. Something that felt like a cannonball hit my forehead just above the bridge of the nose. Red clouds rolled in my skull. My eyes filled with tears. I felt myself being grabbed and swung. I could not see. I flailed with my right arm. The smells of the air were changing from the copilot's sweat and vomit to something bigger, fresher.

The open gondola door.

I grabbed a seat back. He pulled my fingers loose. I could hear the sob of his breath. My vision was clearing. I could see the door, a rectangle of light. I could feel my fingers dragging clear of the seat back. I saw him lean back. He was doing something with his leg, but I was still stunned from the head butt, slow as a glacier. Even slower than him.

He kicked me in the stomach.

I lurched backward into the doorway. I grabbed at the jamb with my left hand. The fingers were still not working. The air out there was cold and fresh. All three thousand feet of it.

I thought: This is not happening.

My fingers skidded off the door jamb.

I fell.

It is true, what they say about your life passing before your eyes. I saw Rhyd and Camilla. And my parents. And the boys. They were all there, for an individual thought, and a goodbye.

Or perhaps it was a hello.

Except for the boys.

I felt terrible about the boys.

I hit something.

I hit it with a thump that knocked all the wind out of me. It was an iron bar. I was draped over it like a clothes peg. So this is what it feels like to die, I thought. It hurts.

I opened my eyes.

All around me was a gray mist. Limbo.

Not limbo. Cloud.

I was draped over the skid of the airship. Next to my arm was the boarding ladder.

The cloud parted for a moment. All the way down there, gray and wrinkled like the skin of a rhino, was the sea.

My fingers found the boarding ladder, clamped on. I got a foot up. I was moving slowly, like an old man with brittle bones. Bones get very brittle when they hit water from a three-thousand-foot cloud base.

My left hand was beginning to work.

There were vibrations in the gondola. Drumbeats. Footsteps. The footsteps were going away, to the left. Walking up the aisle. A door slammed. The door between the cabins. I gripped the ladder. I climbed.

The airship lurched, hitting a pocket of turbulence. My arm muscles cracked. The cloud was cold on my face.

My head came above the level of the sill. There were no feet under the seats. I pulled myself in. The copilot was forward, in his seat. The door in the partition was open. He was slumped in his seat, head in hands. I thought of his green-gray skin, the smell of sweat and vomit. Concussion. Fighting would have weakened him. The airship was sliding back, standing on its tail. The mooring lines were lashing back, writhing like serpents. One of them slapped the windscreen. His hand pawed the aileron wheel. The airship lurched again. I stumbled. The nose was still up, the gangway a steep hill.

He turned his head at me. His face was the color of a stone dug out of subsoil. He brought his right hand up from under the seat. In the hand was an odd-looking gun.

I dived for the floor. It was sloping backward at seventy degrees. My feet were braced against a seat. I shoved the door upward. It slammed.

At the same moment, he fired.

I heard the bang. The cockpit filled with a red glare. The cloud outside glowed the color of blood. The airship bucked like a breaching whale.

I saw the copilot's feet in the dried blood on the partition, the wall that was now a floor. The flare's smoke wreathed in there. I saw his feet shuffle a lurching two-step. I saw them go sideways, across the door to the back of the pilot's seat. Then, through the blood-smeared partition, I saw a thing that drove me to my knees and locked my arms around the solid supports of a seat.

The airship plunged tail-first out of the cloud into clear air. I saw the copilot's feet, uncoordinated by concussion, trip on the pilot's seat and vanish. I saw his arms spread. I saw him fall sideways out of the open pilot's door. I saw the mooring rope writhing out there, his hands grab for it, catch it.

I saw his face.

The face was screwed up with terror. When his hands locked on the rope and the rope took his weight, the terror changed to a relief that smoothed out the lines and furrows so the face was once more the face of a child who did not know about being a foot soldier, or anything except that he was going to grow up, and be fine, and live forever.

I saw the relief turn to terror.

The rope was attached to the nose of the airship. I do not know if he had already hit the switch to fill the fore ballonets, or whether it was his weight that did it.

The nose started to sink.

For a moment he clung to the rope, dangling outside the cabin.

Then he began to swing.

He hung on to the end of the eighty-foot rope as the airship's nose came down and became the focal point of an arc that swung out and across, as lazy and graceful as the trajectory of a trapeze artist, three thousand feet in the air. At the end of the arc, either he had fainted, or his hands would no longer hold the rope.

Either way, he let go.

His body continued the arc upward. For a moment, he looked as if he might fly.

He did not fly.

He fell.

He fell straight down, without struggling. The rope hung limp from the airship's nose.

I did not see him hit the sea, because you cannot see a human figure from a mile in the air. Besides, I was being sick.

I must have lain there for some time. After a while, I found the strength to crawl into the cockpit and fiddle with the ballonet switches until I had the airship trimmed horizontal, descending slowly. Then I went aft into the passenger cabin and dragged the life raft out of its compartment. The gray sea came up to meet me. The wrinkles became a low swell. When we were twenty feet up I heaved the canister out of the door and pulled the release line.

The big yellow doughnut swelled, bloomed and touched the water. It started dragging, towed by the windage of the airship. I unclipped the line, wrapped it around my hand, and jumped. I landed half in, half out of the raft, with a thump that knocked the breath out of me.

When I could breathe, I looked out. The airship was three hundred yards downwind, blowing sideways. Anyone but me would probably have thought it looked beautiful, and gigantic, and ecologically sound.

I turned my head away.

The swell was running six to eight feet. I was cold, and wet, and rolling around the life raft like a cannonball on a flatbed truck.

I could not remember a time when I had been so happy.

I dug in the emergency pack, found an EPIRB, pulled the ring.

They must have been up there looking for me. A very short time later, it seemed, the light was flickering overhead, and there was noise: the hellish *whock* of rotors and the roar of an engine. A helmet bore the words U.S. COAST GUARD. A loop of webbing tightened under my arms. For the second time in four weeks, I ascended into a new world.

And this time I had an admission ticket and I knew the script.

They flew me to hospital in Rockland. A doctor examined me from head to foot. He found nothing wrong except for some bruising to the ribs.

When the doctor had finished, there was a policeman waiting outside. He took me down to the precinct and started to take a statement. I was thinking again now. I was thinking about a list of people of whom I had to ask questions.

The police had some questions of their own. I told them enough to get me out of there, walked down Main Street, rented another car, and told the renters where they could come and fetch it. I was hungry, as long as I did not think of what had happened up there under that gray roof of cloud. I ate two roast beef sandwiches with chopped olives, coleslaw and mustard, and called Ricky Lee. Erin's answering machine said they were both out right now. I left a message. Then I called the *Duchess of Malfi*, and had myself put through to Pierce Rapaport.

The voice on the other end said, "Who shall I say is calling?"

I gave my name. There was a silence. Pierce came on. He said, "Okay, who the hell's that?"

I said, "George Devis."

There was a silence. *"George,"* he said. "Sorry. She told me it was Warren Diglis." He laughed. The laugh ended in a cough. "Cold," he said. "Well, how did it go?"

I said, "Where's Poliakoff?"

"Out of the country."

"When did he leave?"

"This morning."

"In a hurry?"

Pierce laughed. "He's always in a hurry. Did you get a tape out of Ras Hamil?"

I said, "The airship crashed. Everyone survived, except the copilot. You were wrong about Ras Hamil. We were set up. I've got a story for you. A good big one."

He said, sharply, "What kind of story?"

I said, "The kind of story that will make you want to change your boss."

"I see." His voice was guarded now. "Does this have to do with Serge flying out?"

"It does," I said.

Pierce said, "Can you tell me any more right now?"

"Later."

He said, "I'm very grateful to you for this."

I said, "Not at all." I slammed down the receiver and headed north.

The traffic was thickening up. There were a lot of campers, and the Maine Lobster stalls by the roadside were doing big business. After the mall outside Ellsworth I turned right for Bar Harbor. It was five o'clock in the afternoon. The day seemed to have lasted a hundred years. I thought of the first time I had driven up here, the day after the burglary on *Halcyon,* visiting Charis Brown that time, too, with a jarful of hot flour. My eyelids were falling over my eyes and my thoughts were fuzzy and confused. I did not need to be fuzzy and confused. I pulled off the road, leaned my head against the window, and went to sleep.

It was dusk when I woke. I pulled on to the road, drove over the bridge on to Mount Desert Island, through the lit-up Edwardian splendor of Bar Harbor and into the dark country beyond. Cottage windows glowed yellow through the trees by the road. The sky was still blotted out by cloud. I felt achy and dull in the head. But I knew where I was going and what I had to do.

There was a car waiting by the side of the road ahead. I flashed my lights at it. It flashed back. Its high-rumped boot glowed candy-apple red in the headlamps as I pulled in behind.

Ricky Lee climbed out of the Mustang and into the head-lights. I went to meet her. She hung around my neck. She said, "I can't believe you're here."

I was feeling a little light-headed myself. Her hair smelled faintly of perfume. I said, "It's down to you."

She said, "I called Warren Diglis about that guy at the airfield. He said he didn't know anything about him."

I said, "Amazing. Maybe he's lying."

She said, "They working for Poliakoff?"

"That's right." I told her why.

She said, "My Lord." She looked at me with eyes about double their normal size.

"Story for you," I said.

She said, "Something's happening at PKC. The share price went down ten percent in the last hour of trading."

"And Poliakoff's out of the country."

She said, "Why would the share price drop?"

"You tell me," I said.

"News Actuality's been losing money," she said. "The papers break even, I guess. The rest of it, who knows? But why so sudden?"

I said, "Where did he go?"

"Russia, someplace," she said. "Listen, if you think this is a story, you're crazy. You've only got Hamil's word against him, and thanks to you Hamil's got no credibility. Lawyers Poliakoff's got, you're dead."

I laughed. As far as Poliakoff was concerned, I was dead already. I said, "Drive. I'll show you."

She drove. After five miles, she looked at me sideways. "Stories aside," she said, "I'm glad you're back."

I took her hand. I said, "Thank you for bringing the car." Like honeymooners, we turned off the road and into the grove of pines in which stood the house of Charis Brown.

It was a cold night. Light crept out through the chinks in the curtains. I hammered on the door.

"Who's there?" said the big, croaking voice.

I told her. She opened up. She said, "This is a surprise." Her face was gray and coarse, the skin large-pored. There were heavy double bags under her eyes. She looked as if she did not mean it was a nice surprise.

I said, "I think we should talk."

Her eyes became fixed and suspicious. "It's not particularly convenient," she said.

"It's quite urgent," I said.

Her eyes moved across to Ricky Lee. I saw them flick up and down, checking the fit of the jeans, the breasts under the T-shirt. It was a predatory, male sort of once-over. "You'd better come in," she said.

We went into the living room with the grubby Navajo blanket on the floor. My eyes strayed to the bookshelves where she kept *Auks* and the *Best Guide to British Birds* by George Devis.

The books were no longer there.

I said, "I think the time has come for you to be frank, Charis."

Her eyes had followed my eyes. Now they were defensive: the eyes of a set-dresser caught set-dressing. She sighed.

She said, "What exactly is it that you want to know?"

37

*T*HE EMERGENCY RELIEF BUREAU," I SAID. RICKY LEE HAD HER pad out and was writing shorthand. She also had a tape recorder going in her bag, but Charis Brown did not need to know that. "ERB. It's not a government body."

She raised her eyebrows. The bags under her eyes were big and grainy. "Isn't it?"

I said, "The first time we met, you were saying you didn't approve of Serge Poliakoff, because you didn't like to see first-class minds being bought."

She watched me, not moving.

"But he bought yours."

She ducked her head. She said, "I suppose I should be flattered."

"He wanted someone at the UN. You were it."

Her face was hard, and cold, and unmoving. She said, "I helped you out. This is an odd way of paying me back."

I said, "Serge Poliakoff's in big trouble. You're in trouble. They'll spread your life out on a big table and they'll pull it apart and they won't stop till they find something."

She watched me for what felt like five minutes. She went to a cupboard, slopped two inches of Johnny Walker into a glass, and sat down in the brown corduroy armchair. She said, "And you've bust him open." She tipped the whiskey down her throat. "Full immunity?"

I said, "Not my decision. You tell me about the ERB. I'll put in a word, for what it's worth."

She said, "It was all because that damn Caroline Impey wanted to get into your pants. She sent you off to Ohio and you never even called her back." Her voice had turned hard and nasty.

"She told me about the irradiation, and you couldn't stop her, because it would have looked strange. Then she told you that she'd given me Bruno Wanamaker's name."

"Yes."

"And who did you tell?"

She said, "I have the ERB fax number. I don't know any of the people. Sometimes they fax me, ask me to write them a report. They pay me. It's always happened like that."

"How did you know you weren't working for the government?"

"They pay too much."

"What was your connection with Bruno Wanamaker?"

She dropped her eyes. "I'd received a fax requesting advice on the marking of a load of wheat bound for Ethiopia."

"About which we know."

"About which you found out."

"And you didn't want to know why they wanted this information?"

"No."

There was a silence.

"I tried to warn you," she said. "Aid and spooks. You don't ask questions. It's no world for a guy like you." Her mouth turned down at the corners. "Nice. Straightforward."

I said, "We seem to have done all right."

She said, "You were lucky." The maiden aunt had gone.

Now she was a tough, spooky old bureaucrat with her back to the wall.

I said, "Please give me the fax number of the ERB."

She went to a filing cabinet in the corner, pulled out a folder, tore a strip of paper off a fax roll, passed it over. It meant nothing to me. I read it out to Ricky Lee.

"Boston area code," she said.

I got up. "Thank you, Miss Brown," I said.

Her face had gone slack and deadly. She said, "There are always people like you and your damn sister. You think you can change the world. But things work in a certain way. It's a machine, and it exists, and you can't change it or stop it." We were at the door. "I hope your car crashes," she said.

Ricky Lee tucked her notebook away in her handbag. "Why, thank you," she said.

I drove the Mustang back to Bar Harbor. We checked into the Harbor Hotel and walked to Captain Cutler's Lobster Shack by the quay. It was a warm night. We ordered a bottle of white wine. My head felt like a sack of cement. I said, "Can you track a fax number?"

Ricky Lee said, "I'll try tomorrow."

I said, "Fine." The room was spinning.

She said, "You look terrible. Let's get you back to the hotel."

In the hotel room, she got on the telephone. I sat on the bed. Sitting became lying. My head was on the pillow. I passed out.

When I woke up again, she was still on the telephone. She was in her white nightdress, and the sun was pouring in through the window. The clock radio said eleven A.M. She could have been there all night.

When she saw me she came across the floor like a dancer and poured coffee out of the Thermos jug on the bedside table. "You still look terrible," she said with horrid brightness. "I've done real good. I got the owner of the fax. And Ras Hamil was on the answering machine. I called him. He's flying in in twenty minutes."

I stumbled out of bed. The hotel had laundered my clothes. I drank three cups of coffee and shaved with a hand that showed a tendency to shake. Otherwise, I looked as if I had been leading the open-air life, like the other tourists seeping into Bar Harbor for the season.

I went downstairs to the restaurant. There were a couple of yachts at the pontoon outside the window. The day was clear and sunny and the tables on the deck were filling up with early lunchers in polo shirts. I did not like the holiday look of it. I wanted to stay inside, in the gloom, where nobody could see me.

So I found a table in a corner and sat in the angle of the walls under a whaling print, eating eggs and bacon and four slices of brown toast and watching the door. After ten minutes, Ras Hamil came in.

He was with the bodyguard. The bodyguard stayed near the door, towering over the six-foot-three-inch headwaiter. Ras Hamil walked toward me, arms open, lanky in his loose-fitting khaki fatigues. His skin shone in the dark restaurant and his smile cast a beam of light into the dim corners. "George," he said. "My friend." His voice was loaded with warmth. "Are you well? They told me you are well."

He sat down and ordered a glass of water, politely, not at all like a warlord.

I had been thinking. I said, "I owe you an apology."

He thought about that, hard, as if he could not imagine what I was driving at. He said, "Why would this be?"

"I have been very naïve. I was nearly the . . . instrument of your death."

He laughed, a big laugh that had more in common with the holiday people at the tables outside than the dark shadows of the corner. "At home, I have been ambushed," he said. "My house has been bombed. My food has been poisoned. Aircraft in which I am thought to be traveling have vanished. I see these not as crimes, but as . . . outbreaks of practical politics." The eyes were clownish and big, the hands spread, the way they had been spread in the photograph he had showed me on the airship. I found I was laughing, too. Even the bodyguard was grinning, over by the door. There goes the boss, he must be thinking. Ras Hamil had an amazing power of inspiring affection.

He said, "Are you well yourself?"

I said, "I'm fine. The copilot had an accident."

The laughter left his face. Behind it, I caught a glimpse of the toughness he must have needed to stay alive among the guns and bombs and poison. "I see," he said. "I telephoned the pilot in hospital. He was . . . very surprised by what took place. He is recovering. So all is well, I think. In fact, I must thank you for the opportunity we had to meet the people of Matinicus. A lady gave us coffee and cake."

I tried to imagine him and the giant bodyguard and the lacerated pilot with a little old Maine lady in the parlor of a wooden house, making conversation over the coffee cups. It was not a picture that came easily to the mind.

"So that is a thing," he said. "There is another. I have spoken with Jerry Stein in Bristol. He says that since your tour he has the means to put in place another twenty project advisers. The village of Rhyd and Camilla will have its adviser again. For this I thank you."

I said, "I raised the money by slandering you."

He grinned again. He said, "People are less important than change. I am the fulcrum; history is the lever." I thought: Here is a wonderful thing, a politician who does not see himself as the center of the universe. "But there is a last problem," he said. "I did not speak of it yesterday because I thought we might die, and I did not want to speak of the future to a man about to die." He said it as if it was an everyday piece of good manners. For him, it probably was. "I think you spoke of a detailed analysis Rhyd made of the system by which the marked shipment of corn reached him. It would be of great use if you could find this."

I said, "Of course."

"But you do not know where?"

I said, "Not for certain."

Hamil sighed. "So," he said. "It might as well have burned in the house. There is no analysis. There will be a long and dirty unraveling. I must leave for Ethiopia tonight." He held out his hand and laid it on the table; not in the shaking position, but palm up, fingers closed, as if he was hiding something. "And you can think of green villages, and leaves growing back upon the Alleluia Tree."

He opened the fingers. In the palm was a silver cross, massive and barbaric, set with stones the color of a lion's eyes. "Esias your friend made this," he said. "It is my thanks to you and your family. Tell the boys to visit me. Come yourself."

He got up. I was looking at the cross, smelling ashes.

When I looked up, he was gone.

I walked slowly back upstairs. The metal of the cross was warm in my hand. In the room Ricky Lee was writing in a notebook. I sat down in the chair and looked out at the bright harbor and the wide blue gleam of Frenchman Bay.

I thought of the dark valley at Bethel, the crunch of waves, the hiss of the wind in the giant maple in the yard. I thought of the Rhyd tapes, "Birdman in the Corn," the scratch and plink of the clawhammer banjo track, caught like shreds of ribbon in the branches of the first and original Alleluia Tree.

Ricky Lee said, "Oh, no."

She was standing in front of the television, which was switched on, the way people in Europe might light a log fire in summer for something to flicker in the corner.

It was a local news program. There was a picture of a grove of pines and what had once been a brown clapboard house. It was not a house any more. Firemen in big helmets were damping down the rubble, which was still steaming. Before it had caught fire, it had been the residence of Charis Brown.

The newscaster was saying that human remains had been discovered in the wreckage. The freckles were muddy blotches on Ricky Lee's white skin. "They killed her," she said.

"They've killed a lot of people," I said.

I picked up the telephone and dialed the number of the ERB. It rang twice. A woman answered. I said, "This is the Directory Information service of Bell Telephone. I am afraid that due to a computer failure we may have you miscatalogued. Can you please give me your address?"

The woman at the other end said, "I'm sorry, sir, I am not at liberty to divulge this information." She put the phone down.

Ricky Lee said, "Give that here. I'll call the billing department."

I thought about Charis Brown. She would not have told anyone that she had told us. It was likely that whoever had killed her would have done it to keep her quiet, not as an act of revenge.

Ricky Lee and I knew too much as well.

The bedroom was not a bedroom with the sun shining off the sea now. It was a trap, and its air held the distant whiff of death.

Ricky Lee was writing on a pad. She thanked somebody and hung up. "Bills go to Georgetown Investment," she said.

"Can you get a listing? Any further information?"

She nodded. She was avoiding my eye. She said, "If someone killed Charis Brown, they'll want to kill us, right?"

"That's right," I said. "Unless we get to them first."

"How?"

I tried to look reassuring. I said, "Let's find out about Georgetown."

She began telephoning again. I went out of the room. The hallway was empty. There was a telephone at the end. I picked it up, dialed the number of Rooney's Lunch and Lobster in Quogue. Danny answered.

I did not let him gossip. I said, "Is John there?"

"Wait there," he said. "Yeah, sure. He's on his boat. I can see him from—"

"Could you ask him to call me?"

"Sure," he said. "Gimme a number."

I gave him the number of the hotel. "I'll be here for an hour," I said. Then I went back to the room.

Ricky Lee said, "Group of corporations of which Georgetown Investments is a member." She pushed a notebook at me.

I said, "Call a paper that doesn't belong to Poliakoff. Tell someone you have a story."

She started dialing.

The notebook held a list of names. There was the Emergency Resources Bureau, and a lot of other companies I did not recognize. There was also something called Sports Projects.

Sports Projects had a telephone number. I walked down the hall again and called it. I said, "Am I talking to the owners of *Woods and River*?"

"You certainly are," said the voice on the far end. It was not an intelligent voice, which was most satisfactory.

"And you do some fight promoting, right?"

"Through Fistic," said the voice. "Can I put you through?"

"And a fishing fleet?"

"We own some boats," said the voice.

"Scallop dragging?" I was remembering Bill in *Auk's* cockpit, in the fog, without a head.

"How did you *know?*" said the voice.

"I have a great research department," I said.

"Why do you *want* to know?" said the voice.

"I was thinking of taking you over," I said.

"Oh," said the voice, worried now. "I don't . . ."

"Joke," I said. I put the telephone down.

Sullivan had edited the Boston *Echo*. The owner of *Woods and River* had known of his piscatorial ambitions and given him a new job to make him forget about anything Bill might tell him. When I had visited Bruno Wanamaker, the upscale Eastern Midwestern hayseed, he had called the owner of ERB. And Warren Diglis had no doubt owed favors to Fistic, and would have supplied its owner with muscle on demand.

I walked back to the room.

Ricky Lee said, "A reporter'll call back." The telephone rang. She picked it up, frowned. "For you," she said.

It was John. "You okay?" he said.

"Fine."

"Messages at Rooney's," said John. "Couple of reporters. One weird one."

"Oh yes?"

"Guy with a Southern accent, Danny says," said John. "Made Danny write it down. Pissed Danny off. He don't write so well."

"Read it," I said.

"It says: 'Take a ticket back to England. Boys happy at Bethel, because they're still with us. One move from you, and they go join Daddy.'"

I stood there with my heart pumping iced water instead of blood.

"Oh, yeah," John said. "Guy had a cold, Danny said."

I said, "I know." There was a long, humming silence. I said, "We need a fast boat, long range."

"Sure," said John. "Going where?"

I told him. He said, "Be on the town dock in Northeast Harbor in two hours."

I put the telephone down.

It rang again immediately. "Hi," said an eager reporterish voice. "Can I speak with Ricky Lee Klaasen?"

"She's not here," I said, and put the receiver down.

Ricky Lee said, "Hey!"

"Change of plan," I said.

"What?"

"Book me a ticket to England through a Poliakoff company, flying tomorrow. I'll pack the bags."

"Ticket?"

"Please."

She stared at me. She opened her mouth to say something, but she saw something in my face that made her change her mind. She shrugged. I packed. Half an hour later, we checked out.

Mount Desert Island is famous for its scenery. I did not notice any of it as we drove to Northeast Harbor. I was thinking that Poliakoff might have taken off for Russia with his share price dropping like a brick, but that he still had a machine, and that he had left the machine in motion.

Hamil was flying out. But I and Ricky Lee were caught up in the gears.

And so were the boys.

John was waiting on the dock. He looked reassuringly big. The day was dazzlingly clear and hot. He was wearing a heavy plaid shirt and khaki shorts. He said, "Got your boat," and gestured over the lip of the quay.

A thirty-five-foot lobster boat was nuzzling the piles. It was a work-eroded brute, with a big well and the battered relics of a wheelhouse. "GMC V8 truck engine, turbocharged," he said. "Won the Quogue Derby last year. Do twenty knots, easy."

"Extra diesel?"

"Everything you need." His eyes glittered above his beard.

I said to Ricky Lee, "Down you go." I followed her down the ladder. John came after me. He twisted the key. The engine started with a roar like five trucks in a tin shed. I cast off. John rammed the throttle halfway up and spun the wheel. White foam boiled under the counter and the deck surged forward. Ricky Lee wrinkled her nose at the strong smell of long-dead bait.

We threaded our way out through the lobster boats. John shoved the throttle on to the stop. The lobster-claw nose of the boat lifted and settled on to a cushion of whizzing spray.

The hammer of the engine was a solid object as we towed a vee of wake out of the harbor. There were gulls, and loons, and duck skittering for cover across the waves. I paid them no attention. I was thinking about the boys, in that black and foggy valley.

And in my mind, the line of Rhyd's song was running. It was

C L A W H A M M E R

a version of my own, clawhammer banjo, Rhyd's voice over the top:

When the Book of Life is written
To which this is the key,
The Lord will post in the library
By the Alleluia Tree.

38

*T*HE AFTERNOON TURNED INTO A LONG, MONOTONOUS HAMMER across a sea made of chips of sapphire. John had brought some cold barbecued chicken and poppyseed rolls from the bakery in Red Hill. Ricky Lee ate. I was not hungry. I was sitting on an upturned bucket, watching the wake spew out from under the stern.

At seven o'clock the sun was still high in the sky and the air was clear as spring water. The branches of the black pines on the rocks were tipped with new green. Beyond the maniac clatter of the engine, birds were undoubtedly singing. It was going to be a beautiful evening.

John was pointing ahead. Across the green heave of the sea, a narrow white finger jutted against a far black promontory. I glanced at the chart. Butcher Island light. These were the charts from *Halcyon*. We had used them the last time we had been in, following Rhyd's pencil spider marks. They had been reassuring then. They were less reassuring now. Things were running too fast, out of control.

John pulled back the revs. The nose of the boat sank into its white pillow of foam. We churned between the narrowing shores of the bay. I told John what I wanted him to do. I said, "He goes armed."

He grinned at me. He said, "As a licensed dope dealer, I guess I seen worse than him."

We nosed into the stony cove we had used last time, dropped the anchor. I heaved the little Avon inflatable over the side.

I said to Ricky Lee, "Stay here."

She nodded. She looked white and frightened.

John climbed into the dinghy. I pulled us ashore and hid it in the pines at the top of the beach. We walked around and over the headland. From the spine of the rocks, the roof of Chuck's barn was a sharp horizontal among the trees. The breeze hissed in the leaves of the maples by the burying ground.

I pointed out the barn to John.

He grinned out of the fastnesses of his beard. It was a new kind of grin. I thought there might be relief in it, as if he was at long last getting a chance to return some of the favors Rhyd had done him. Then he set off along the beach at a fast, ungainly lope, rattling pebbles.

I let him get a hundred yards ahead. Then, quietly, I began to pick my way over the stones and driftwood in his wake.

When I was halfway down the beach, I heard a noise. It was a big hammering, wood on wood. John, knocking on a door with a log. It went on for a couple of minutes, then stopped abruptly. I kept walking.

The door opened. A voice out of sight above my head said, "What you want?" It was a slow voice, blurred at the edges. Chuck's voice.

John's voice said, "Sir, I am a visitor here. I need information, direction. Maybe hospitality."

"Private property," said Chuck. "Go away. I got a gun."

Scotch John kept talking. "Sir, buddy, I would go away if I could. But I do not know the way to away, if you take my meaning. Maybe you could show me how to get out of here?"

Chuck said, "I'll git you on the road."

"The road?" said John. "Oh, excellent, sir. Because I have a weakness. Left to myself, I tend to steal things."

"Steal?" said Chuck. "Wait." I heard his feet thump in the barn. I heard him come back to the door.

"Oh, sir," said John. "Can this be a firearm?"

"It's a gun," said Chuck. He sounded flustered. "Now git in the truck. I don't like thiefs."

I was not listening to the voices. I was listening to a sound behind the voices. Among the trees' sigh and the crunch of the surf and the muted chorus of birds was another sound. The faint scratch-chicka, scratch-chicka of a clawhammer banjo.

I waited for the truck to start and die away. Then I scrambled up the bank.

The door in the barn's gable end was shut. I tried the handle. It gave. I walked in.

The living room was much the same as before. A rifle lay in pieces on the workbench. There was a smell of oil; Chuck had been cleaning his toys for the hunting season, a mere four months away. I looked at the cassettes. Perfect order, numbered from one to twenty-eight.

I stopped, held my breath.

Through the quiet barn it came, like the clink of a tin heart. *Scratch-chicka.*

From upstairs.

I went up the spiral stairs, very quietly. The noise upstairs continued: two drumlike whacks of fingers across banjo strings, the pluck of the thumb on the top string. Frailing. Clawhammer. A tune was coming out of it. The skeleton of a fiddle tune, played old-time string-band style. It might have been "Cripple Creek."

I was in Chuck's bedroom. Rhyd was grinning at me from the poster on the wall, his eyes chips of light in the dark shadow under his Ace Logging hat.

Scratch-chicka.

From upstairs.

But there were no more stairs.

I tapped the walls. They sounded like wood.

The music was faint, but there, as if it was inside my head. *Scratch-chicka.*

CLAWHAMMER

I opened the wardrobe door. There was the suit, the baseball jacket on hangers, a collection of caps, a smell of sweat.

The noise was louder.

I stood there and listened, and stared at the blank wooden back of the wardrobe.

The not-quite-blank wooden back of the wardrobe.

On the right-hand side was a dark patch. The kind of patch you get if you push with oily hands. Hands that might be oily from the perpetual cleaning and handling of guns.

Scratch-chicka.

I reached out my right hand and pushed the boards.

The back of the cupboard swung away from me.

There was another spiral staircase. At the top of the spiral staircase there was a room.

It was a small room, with walls that leaned in, following the slope of the mansard roof into which it was built. It was painted whitish, and lit by two skylights in the flatter top slope of the roof, so they would be hard to see from outside. On the walls were pictures cut out of magazines: pictures of people with big smiles and bigger hats, dressed in rhinestones and fringes and anteater-hide boots with Mexican heels. Rhyd was there. So were Willie Nelson, Bill Monroe, Wynona Judd, the Seldom Scene, Gram Parsons, Loretta Lynn, Emmylou Harris, Sneezy Waters, the Kentucky Colonels and maybe fifty more.

On the floor was a carpet, blue and white striped. On the carpet was a bed with a patchwork quilt, also blue and white, fresh and zingy in the light from the sun. It was a teenage girl's room, neat and tidy and full of happiness, reached by a spiral staircase behind a secret door.

In the bed under the quilt was a woman. She had a mass of blond hair, spread on three pillows. Her face was bent over to one side, as if the bones of her neck were twisted. The nose was a bony hatchet, the cheekbones two anvils from which the drum-tight skin ran across emaciated hollows to her jawbone. The right cheek was pressed into the pillow. If she had been looking straight ahead, she would have been looking at my feet.

But her eyes were looking up at me, cranked sideways as far as they could go. She was smiling, a most beautiful smile.

Her right arm outside the quilt rested on the pot of an old banjo. The clawed fingers moved over the strings.

Scratch-chicka.

She made a noise in her throat. One of the fingers pointed at the wall. There was a group of pictures up there. They were all of the same blond woman, surrounded by fringes and heels, herself wearing jeans and cowboy boots, smiling a smile that was not the showbiz rictus of the country musicians, but a real smile.

The smile on the face in the bed.

I said, "Hello, Maria."

The hand left the banjo. It came slowly over the quilt, as if it was a great weight. It settled over the table by the bed. There were photographs on the table, a stereo tape deck. The hand hung over the photographs; pointed to one. Rhyd, Camilla, me and the ducks. Behind it was one of her with Ricky Lee, on a stage, singing harmony.

I said, "That's right." I went and took her hand. She smiled and smiled, and made the noise in her throat, and moved her hand from side to side, because it was the only thing she could do.

She let go of my hand. With great effort, she dabbed with her fingers under the pillow. She smiled. I slid in my fingers. It was cool in there. There was something hard and rectangular. A cassette case.

She took it, slotted it dextrously into the machine. I got the feeling it was one of the last things her body would still do well, and she wanted to show me.

A faint hiss came from the big speakers on the walls. A voice came from the speakers. Rhyd's voice. There was no backing track. It said, "This is Rhydian Walters. This recording is an affidavit concerning the linked activities of Eugene Wollo of the Sudanese Police and the Emergency Resources Bureau, apparently a subsidiary of Poliakoff Communications, based in Boston, U.S.A. It deals with an attempt by the Emergency

Resources Bureau to subvert the democratic process in an emerging democracy by means including misappropriations, coercion and fraud. There is an introduction, a précis, and final notes referring to consignment numbers and correspondence. I have included witnesses' statements as and when germane . . ."

My heart was going like a riveting gun. I said, "Could I take a copy of this?"

She signaled yes with her hand. There was a damp patch under her eyes on the pillows. I dried her eyes. I sat there and held her head while she wept. I felt like weeping myself. I remembered what Ricky Lee had said, the night I had found her breaking into my car: *She drank. She couldn't find the strings any more.*

But it had not been drink. It had been the early signs of what looked like motor neurone disease. She had left her friends, and thrown herself on the mercy of her sister.

Some mercy.

I went and started the tape copying on Chuck's machine. The machine Rhyd had sent it to, knowing that Chuck would store it in his library but not be interested, so Bill could go and track it down, primed by his last homemade tape from Ethiopia. Not knowing that Chuck would share it with his sister, who would treasure every word, because it was a voice from outside the four walls of her room.

Most of it dealt with Ethiopia. The names were names I had heard mentioned, but they meant little, so I skipped that part. The part of particular interest was the part that dealt with the ownership of the ERB, apparently a subsidiary of Poliakoff Communications.

Apparently.

When I had listened to it, I slipped it into my pocket. It clicked against the silver cross Esias had made for Ras Hamil. *In the name of my sister, and of God,* I thought. I told Maria I would be back, went down the stairs, walked under the Alleluia Tree and across to the house.

The yard was empty. Flies buzzed in the patches of sun that

crept through the branches of the tree, and a pig clanked a bucket in the sty. There was an unpleasant fluttering in my stomach as I walked up the steps and knocked on the door of the house.

There were footsteps, quick and exasperated. The door opened. It was Sarah; a Sarah pale and haggard, wisps of hair trailing from her bun. She looked as if she had not slept for several days. When she saw me her eyes snapped wide. She said, "Oh, no."

I said, "I've come for the boys."

She said, "No, you haven't. Not yet. I've just had them on the phone."

"Had who on the phone?"

"Your lawyers. They've secured a court order. They'll be down here in an hour. Less than an hour. And let me tell you, we'll be looking very closely at your court order, me and the lawyers from Greenbank. It's not only the world and the flesh that has the law—"

I said, "I haven't called any lawyers. I don't know what you're talking about."

She stopped in mid-sentence. Her mouth was open.

I said, "There is no injunction, or court order, or whatever you call it."

She said, "But he called. A man. He's coming. He said he was your lawyer."

I said, "He's lying."

"Then . . ."

I said, "I've just met your sister Maria."

A red tide of blood rose from her neck to her forehead. She said, "Where's Chuck?"

"Chasing someone off the property. Now I'd like to come in."

Her eyes were lowered. She nodded, and led me into the parlor. We sat on the hard ladder-backed chairs. The sacred embroideries looked blandly down. She said, "You don't understand."

I said, "I think I do."

"You couldn't."

I said, "I'll try."

She raised her eyebrows and folded her hands in an attitude of strained piety. I thought of the crossings-out in the family Bible. I went on.

"Rhyd jumped ship," I said. "Rejected the Brethren, so you tell yourself he doesn't exist for you. But he exists for Chuck. Chuck is God's punishment on you because you loved Rhyd, and you still do. So Chuck is a just punishment.

"Maria was different. She was out there with the band, singing the Devil's tunes. Then she started to get a little shaky, lost control of her left hand. People thought she was drinking. Actually, she was showing early signs of motor neurone disease. So you took her in here. She's still got a one hundred percent mind, but you locked her away in an attic without a door, with a staircase she couldn't climb in a million years, to reflect on the punishment your God handed out to her. You told everyone she was dead. Including Rhyd. That was, what, four years ago? He hadn't seen you since. Which I think is the only reason he didn't change the guardianship clause in his will. Maybe you were a good sister to Rhyd once. Maria's illness changed you. Right?"

"It is the vengeance of the Lord," she said. "It was His sign that we had erred and strayed as a family."

"So you turned back to the straight and narrow," I said. "And you're waiting for her to die. Clutching those sins to your bosom, Sarah. You're telling yourself you're carrying the burden of your sins and Maria's sins. But there's something else."

She raised her gray eyes. They held cold flames of anger. She said, "What would that be?"

"Not very noble," I said. "Something like, Not-in-front-of-the-neighbors, I guess. Or maybe, Not-in-front-of-the-Brethren. Good old What-will-they-say."

She was still staring at me. But the anger in her eyes was

changing. She was not used to people facing her down or pointing things out to her about herself. Now, she looked as much haunted as angry.

"I have to tell you," I said. "I want the boys back. The Sarah Ebden Rhyd wanted the boys to know is not the woman I'm talking to. I want you to resign your guardianship."

She said, "It is my sacred duty."

I said, "There are two ways of looking at it. One is that you will hand them over to me and sign the release. The other is that I tell the press and the lawyers that you have kept your sister a prisoner for nearly four years, denied her medical attention. I don't think they'll judge you a fit person to exercise care and control over minors." I took a deep breath to slow the thunder of my heart. "There is a quiet way. And there is a noisy way. Which do you want, Sarah?"

The haunted look was gone. The skin around the eyes was gray and twitching. She said, "You still don't understand."

My heart sank.

"I have been vouchsafed a sign. It is my duty to keep these children and do everything in my power to remove them from your influence."

I said, "You are going to regret this."

She said, "In following God's orders, there is nothing to regret."

I said, "There is another thing. The man who rang and said he was my lawyer. He and his people will take the boys away if I do not do as he asks."

"God's will be done."

I sat and watched her and wondered how I had ever thought she was anything but a maniac. I said, "These people who are coming are very dangerous. They wish the boys harm. They killed your brother Rhyd."

She said again, "God's will be done."

I said, "If you won't let them come of their own free will, I'll take them."

She did not say, God's will be done. She started to cry. She said, "You're on a fast train to hell, and you want to take those poor innocents along. You're telling lies to get your evil way."

I said, "You and I are co-guardians." I was panicking. She was drifting. "I want them away from here."

She said, "No."

I looked at my watch. It was nine o'clock. There was very little time. I said, "I'll go and get them."

She started screaming.

As I went out of the room, the sweat was pouring off me. The house seemed full of jagged shadows where there should not have been shadows. It stank of centuries of people twisting their minds into attitudes in which they could believe in things they knew not to be true.

I roared, "Boys!"

I heard an answering shout, quickly shut off. It came from the back of the house, in the wing with the boys' bedrooms. I went down there quickly. There was a passage with a bedroom door on either side, a door at the end of the passage. I heard a key turn in a lock.

I ran the last three steps and hit the door above the lock with the flat of my shoe. There was a crash as the screws tore out of the pine doorpost. The door slammed open.

Joe and Harry were standing against the end wall. Two deacons in their buttoned-up white nylon shirts and charcoal-gray trousers were standing between me and them. I said, "Hello, my dears. Time we were off."

I walked between the deacons. I was entirely calm now. I said, "We've got to go."

The deacons' hands were curled on their upper thighs. They said, "No."

A voice from the doorway said, "Let him."

I turned. Sarah was standing in the center of the doorway, bolt upright in her floral overall. Her face was gray, as if hacked from stone, except around the eyes, where the muscles were wriggling like things in a pond.

"Let him take them out," she said. "He is allowed to see

them." There were other words she was leaving unsaid. *He has no car. Chuck is out there. Chuck has the means to defend his mother, his land, his religion.*

The deacons let their hands fall back to their sides. I felt the boys' hands in mine, one each side. Looking neither right nor left, I led them through the house and into the yard under the green-and-white coins of light that crept through the branches of the Alleluia Tree. They hung on tight. Neither of them said a word.

Any minute now, Chuck was going to be back. I said, "There's a lobster boat anchored past the headland." They nodded. Their eyes were swiveling, terrified. "Ricky Lee's on it. Get around there and get out to the boat. There's a dinghy in the trees. Go."

They started away for the end of the barn, running. I thought: Whatever happens, they'll be all right now.

An engine roared on the track. A Lincoln Continental bounced into the yard on twanging springs.

The car stopped.

The window went down. Something that looked like a black snorkel came out of the window. A voice roared. "Nobody move!"

The thing was not a snorkel. It was a gun.

And the voice was the last voice I wanted to hear.

Even if I had expected to hear it.

39

I TURNED AROUND AND RAISED MY HANDS FROM MY SIDES TO SHOW I was not holding a gun. I moved so I was between the car window and the boys. There was the trunk of the tree, too. They were running. They must be around the end of the barn by now.

The car door opened. The driver got out, the round eye of the gun unwavering between my own two eyes. It looked like Chuck was going to get beaten to it.

I wondered what happened to wards of joint guardians when one was unfit and the other was dead. I hoped it was nothing bad.

I said, "Hello, Pierce."

He smiled. His white Ivy League teeth gleamed in the sun, and his clever eyes twinkled, and so did the chains on his Gucci loafers. He said, "Where are your nephews?"

I said, "I don't know." The gun in his hand was not just a pistol. It looked like the kind of gun that held more cartridges than that and fired them faster. I said, "What's that gun?"

"Heckler and Koch," he said. "Long-range chainsaw. I'll use it, too. Where are the boys?"

I said, "This is a two-hundred-acre farm. They're kids. They could be anywhere."

"So," he said. "You didn't make it in time." He was smiling. Keep going, boys, I thought.

I shrugged. I said, "I'm afraid I wasn't . . . on the ball."

He smiled the old white smile. Above the barrel of the gun, it looked cold-eyed and patronizing.

I said, "Emergency Resources Bureau. A Rapaport corporation."

He said, "Mr. Poliakoff had the great advantage of the Second World War. He got himself recognized as officer material, cornered the Northern European penicillin supply. It was a springboard. You don't find springboards like that nowadays."

"So you have to build your own."

"Correct."

"So Poliakoff's doing the usual corporate dirty work, and under cover of that you're doing even dirtier work. You were riding on his back, sending corn to Gugsa and his friends because they'd promised you mineral licenses in return for arms. And Ras Hamil was saying bullshit to all that. So you marked some corn and you sent it out to find out how Ras Hamil was getting his information. And you sent Gugsa's boys sniffing around with a Geiger counter. And when they found some on Rhyd and Camilla, you knew that they were getting too close to you. So Gugsa's boys shot them and framed Hamil. They would have liked to kill Hamil too, but he had so much popular support they didn't dare."

"Third World countries are dangerous places," said Pierce.

"For you," I said. "Sullivan drops the fact that Bill's got evidence of something, Bill hasn't told him exactly what. He's bringing it back. So you tell a scallop dragger the Argos position and you sink my boat—but I get away. Sullivan is a drunk, but up there in the fog department he has an inkling that all may not be pleasant for him if he is withholding evidence. You give him his dream job on *Woods and River* to get him off the *Echo,* so he's off the case, and what Bill sent home isn't his business any more. But I said some things to him that reactivated the idea he will be acting all illegal if he withholds evidence Bill sent home. To cover his ass, he calls you, and you say you will take care of things, and you call Diglis to send around Jackson to take the tape away from me. But Jackson makes a mess of it."

"I've come for the boys," said Pierce. "I will trade the boys for all copies of any information you have."

"Do me a favor," I said. "I have put a lot of effort into this. Poliakoff told me he had some kind of leverage over Diglis. I think Fistic had leverage over him, too. You used it to get Diglis to frighten me off whenever I looked like getting close to hard information. Bill had been after Poliakoff in Ethiopia. I had the idea he had been after Hamil. Nice for you. The more they came after me, the hotter I roared against Hamil. You set me up like a coconut shy, Pierce."

He smiled. It was the smile of someone who has been the cleverest boy in the class for so long that nobody else impresses him any more. "It wasn't only you I was setting up."

I said, "Poliakoff?"

"I've sold half a million shares short while they dropped forty percent. You and that stupid airship made me ten million dollars."

"Loyalty."

He shrugged, "He was on the slide."

"They'll find you," I said. "They always do." I was looking at the gun, thinking: He is going to rip my head off with that thing and take the boys away. Sarah will drop the case, give him the Rhyd tapes to get them back. There is nothing I can do.

"Not because of anything you tell them," he said. "I'm afraid you won't be around."

The house door crashed open. Sarah came out with the deacons. "Where are the kids?" she said. "Where's Chuck?" Her hair was all the way out of her bun. Her eyes were wild as a hare's. They focused on me. She said, "That's not your car. You came in a boat."

Pierce was quick. He worked out the implications fast. He

stepped back. "Bunch up," he said. "Real close. Now you all trot to the beach with me. Stay in front. I want to speak with those boys."

"Why?" said Sarah. There was a whimper in her voice. Suddenly things were not making sense to her. "Why?"

"They're going to stay with me," he said. "You can collect them later." He had the gun pointed loosely at the group of us. He was smiling politely, reasonable as hell. "Between you, you know rather a lot. I have a big stake in you staying quiet."

I said, "He's killed at least four people. He's going to kill us all. And Chuck. And the boys."

Sarah stared at me, then at him.

He said, "Move."

She jumped at him. She was screaming. "Not Chuck!"

Pierce had not expected this. Middle-aged women with religious mania did not dive at your eyeballs, nails out. Perhaps for a moment something chivalrous stirred in his Ivy League soul. Whatever the reason, he did not rip her in half with his gun. Instead, he reached out his left hand and caught her by the front of the dress. She hung on to the end of his arm. The gun hand did not waver.

Over his shoulder, a movement caught my eye. The thing that had moved was a blotchy red-and-white face with a sunburnt nose under a blue baseball cap. It belonged to an ungainly figure waddling through the trees beyond the yard gates. Chuck.

Chuck stopped. He seemed to be looking carefully at what was happening in the yard. The careful look seemed to last for an hour. Actually, it occupied the time it took Pierce to say, "Be quiet."

Something metallic gleamed in the low sun where Chuck was standing. I was not seeing well. The reddish evening light was interfering with the shadows again, bringing out the red in Pierce's grinning gums, as if his mouth were full of blood that was leaking between his teeth. I thought: This is how vampires look, gorged with blood.

CLAWHAMMER

Somewhere there was an explosion. A hole appeared between the lapels of Pierce's houndstooth jacket, in the middle of his blue-and-white-striped shirtfront. And it was true that he was full of blood, because blood spilled out of his chest and his mouth in two horrible torrents, and he fell forward, taking Sarah down with him.

And from the gate Chuck came running. "Mommy!" he was yelling. "I shot the bad man!"

But his mother did not answer.

Chuck stood there. He started to cry.

I went and pulled Rapaport off her. He was not breathing. Sarah was covered in blood. I took Chuck's rifle gently away from him. Then I looked over her carefully.

It was not all Rapaport's blood. Chuck's Mannlicher was a powerful rifle, and he used solid bullets. Sarah's blood was oozing from a hole in her right shoulder. But she was still breathing.

The fatter of the two deacons seemed to know about first aid. He knelt by the bodies. The other one was talking to Chuck, soothing him. The exclusivity of the Brethren closed over them like the hatch of a tank.

I walked into the house and telephoned for some ambulances. Then I went into Chuck's barn and up the secret stairs and sat by the bed of Rhyd's sister Maria.

Her eyes were rolling wildly, her right hand flapping. I said, "There's been a fight out there. That's what all the noise was. Everyone's fine. We're going to take you to a hospital and they'll look after you. Your friend Ricky Lee will keep you company. Then you can come back, if you want."

The eyes became still, focused on me. She smiled. It was a beautiful smile, like Camilla's.

I said, "Wait a minute." I got up, went down the stairs and onto the beach.

The lobster boat was out there, hovering close inshore, the low sun picking out every fleck of rust and flake of paint. I waved.

The boat came in until it was hanging in the jade green water twenty feet off the beach. John throttled the engine down to a burble. I said, "It's over. Ricky Lee?"

John rowed her ashore in the dory. She was looking at me as if she could see something new in my face; something she was not able to interpret. I grinned at her. She grinned back, tentatively.

John said, "I guess the boys don't like to go ashore again. I'll go see they don't take the boat apart." He pulled back.

I took Ricky Lee up the beach and into the barn. There was the sound of a banjo again, from the top room.

Scratch-chicka.

She said, "Who's here?"

I told her.

She ran up the stairs. I followed her, slowly. When I got to the top, she was sitting on the bed holding Maria's hand in a grip that whitened her knuckles. They were both smiling. They were both crying.

After a while, Ricky Lee turned to me. She said, "I'll go with her."

I nodded. I walked down the stairs into Chuck's room. I went to the Dexion shelves with LIBRY scrawled in red paint. I pulled the Country Cousins tape from its slot and shoved it into the player. Rhyd began singing. I went out of the door, leaving it open.

Beyond the yard, the sun was going down. It poured fire between the leaves of the big maple. The world became a big, sliding blur of red and green. I could not see the terrible thing under the sheet in the yard. And I could not hear the sirens of the ambulances, because Rhyd's voice was there, Camilla singing a high harmony, dobro and guitar, bass, strings and drums, soaring out of the window, sweetening the small, bitter world of the Brethren.

> There were blood-red flowers blooming
> On the Alleluia Tree.

CLAWHAMMER

The song ended. I left the tape hissing, walked out of the yard and on to the beach, into the clean salt smell of the sea.

Harry was standing on the wheelhouse roof. The sun glinted off a pair of binoculars he was training on me. Joe appeared, probably from the bowels of the engine. I waved. They waved back.

John throttled up. The engine began to clatter. A pair of eider ducks flopped away across the water. The boat's forefoot crunched on the beach. I climbed aboard. John shoved the wheel over, and we thundered into the darkening east.